The F*cking

Yoga . . . for The Rest of Us.

by

J. C. Lynne

Ngano Press
www.nganopress.com

Revision 1.0

Trade Paperback
ISBN-10:1-940421-06-3
ISBN-13:978-1-940421-06-3

eBook
ISBN-10:1-940421-09-8
ISBN-13:978-1-940421-09-4

Audiobook
ISBN-10:1-940421-10-1
ISBN-13:978-1-940421-10-0

Cover art by Lillie Fischer

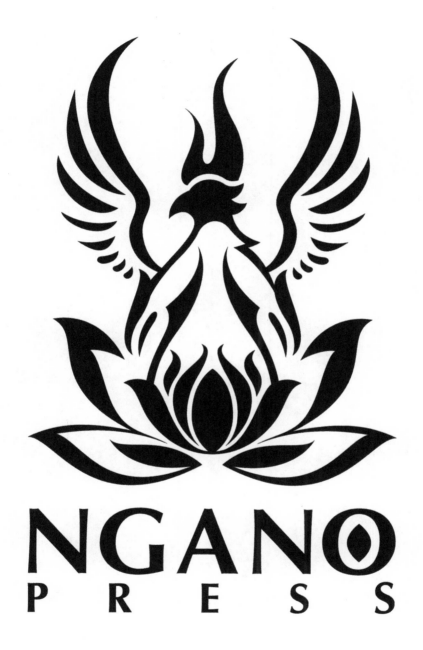

NGANO
PRESS

ACKNOWLEDGEMENTS

I'd like to thank Pam, my first yoga teacher, for inspiring my lifelong passion for yoga; Michael Dillon, affectionately known as The Beard, for the most significant gift anyone has given me, the kick in the ass to do something with my writing (even though he doesn't attend my yoga classes cuz the teacher is a bitch); Courtney Hendrickson Luce, paging Dr. Luce, my friend, colleague, and writing partner who never fails to look at one of my manuscripts and say, "God, that's a beautiful thing"; River Cummings for being both supremely Zen AND down to earth thus making room for this sarcastic bitch to embrace Viniyoga as it works for me; April J. Moore for reading the book with critical eye as a Kriya practitioner, as a talented editor, and with understanding humor; Ronda No H Simmons for providing a different perspective so I could write the best book possible. Sincerest thanks to the Dotter and SIL for producing the audio book during the Covera and protests and general unrest that has been 2020.

Thank you to all of my yoga clients who dig what I'm laying down and have found their passion for yoga.

AUTHOR'S NOTE

I finished this writing this book in 2016. It floated around a bit, changed a bit, and sat a little bit. The manuscript took on its final shape at the beginning of 2020. We were all doing our own thing, hitting the gym, the studio, and recreation centers without a care in the world. You're either reading this book smack in the middle of the global Covid-19 outbreak, and if you're like me, you've been at home for a while . . . a long while. Or you could be reading this book after we've managed to get to post-Covera with a new normal. I don't know what that looks like yet.

Personally, I survived the Rona by hook and crook, I'm a poster child for wear your mask, Bitches! I don't want another round, and I don't want anyone else to drown in their bodily fluids. It's not a pleasant feeling.

At this moment in the continuum, I'm exclusively teaching online, so all of the references to finding a class, going to a studio, or practicing yoga in a community are relevant to our beforetime lives. Particularly in the chapter "As Seen on TV." If you're participating in a lifestyle focused on keeping everyone safe, wearing a mask, limiting your social contact, and resisting the urge to take a blowtorch to someone, in that case, there are very few options EXCEPT video, streaming, or remote yoga.

On a positive note, this makes joining ME online for my brand of yoga a viable option in the Covera wherever you happen to live!

Keeping you safe, keeping me safe, AND keeping our groove on!

J.C. Lynne

September, 2020

https://theeffingyogablog.com/

CHAPTER 1

Fuck That Noise

If you're anything like me, yoga calls to mind Birkenstocks, granola, and Patchouli oil. Frankly, there is no shortage of that kind of vibe in yoga.

If you hate yoga, you are not a monster. Let me say that again so I know you hear me. It's perfectly okay to hate yoga. There is nothing wrong with you.

Sure, there are a ton of different brands of yoga with a variety of gimmicks to appeal to one audience or another, but for the most part, if you are a beginner, yoga bites. Hell, even if you aren't a novice, yoga can suck. I know. I've been practicing yoga for almost thirty-five years and I've been teaching it for nearly sixteen. Yes, I am that old. And I have met MANY types of yoga I don't like.

A lot of people reluctantly attend yoga classes for different reasons. Maybe a doctor recommended it. Or perhaps one thinks it will be a long stretchfest. A therapist might have suggested it to combat stress. Maybe someone is trying to recover from [insert injury here]. Not sleeping? Try yoga. High blood pressure? Try yoga. Feeling stressed and overwhelmed? Fuck it, try yoga. Want to change your career to become a contortionist? Friggin' yoga, baby. Lost a bet? You fucking know it, try yoga. Sound familiar?

More often than not, in pursuing my own yoga, I have found myself in classes with a range of teachers asking clients to do unhealthy things. After listening to my rants about my yoga experiences, classes I've taken, and clients I've had, my husband said, "You're a writer and a yoga instructor. Why don't you write a yoga book?!"

In fairness, he has said it multiple times. The most recent mention elicited a wine-fueled, irritated response, "FINE! I WILL write a book. I'll write a fucking yoga book, and I'm going to call it The Fucking Yoga Book!" If you've picked up this book, you may appreciate the versatility of the word *fuck* as much as I do.

You are reading because something in the depths of your soul giggled at the idea that yoga might actually suck a little. Or you may have had a terrible yoga experience. Yoga may not be your thing. I get it. Just be aware of these truths: You do not have to be flexible to start a yoga practice; you can do yoga at ANY weight and at ANY fitness level; you do not have to be spiritual or in need of transformation (physical or emotional) to do yoga; and you don't have to learn a new language.

It's been my experience that yoga instructors are generally young, slim, and hyper flexible. Yes, I hate them a tiny smidge. I might have been young when I started yoga, but never have I been thin or excessively flexible. I took my first yoga class by accident.

The summer before my senior year in high school, I wrecked my knee waterskiing. Back then, only elite athletes had access to arthroscopic surgery. I managed to keep up with my activities with the help of an unending supply of Ace bandages and athletic tape. Sexy!

When I made the move to university, imagine my horror when I discovered I would have to take a physical education class to graduate. I didn't have a math requirement, but I had a physical education requirement. Whose dumb idea was that? Don't get me wrong; I used to run. I had played tennis since I was six years old. I was a dancer. But gym class? Dodge ball, floor hockey, and flag football weren't high on my list of favorites. Out of all of my choices, yoga seemed like the most innocuous option. I trudged into that yoga class over thirty years ago, ready to pooh-pooh it.

At that time, yoga was still rocking the leotard, the sitar, and the Swami Satchidananda[1] kind of vibe, but hell, anything to get me out of gym class! Thank goodness yoga pants hadn't been invented yet.

---

1   Swami Satchidananda is also known as the "Woodstock Guru" but I would call him the "tiger sex cult" guru. His organization is now mired in a sex scandal involving his compound known as Yogaville. We're talking fraud, sex abuse, and vows of obedience. Not my scene, I have problems with authority.

Pam, the instructor in that long-ago class, was a former nurse who had ruptured several discs caring for a patient. She had seen the horrific results of back fusion and other "corrective" surgeries. Rather than go down that road, she researched non-surgical ways to stabilize her spine. Yoga became her therapy of choice. Something about her method, something about the class, or something about the place in the space-time continuum, resonated for me. I was hooked.

Yoga became my thing. I've been practicing ever since, and began teaching yoga in 2005.

Yoga allowed me to continue to run and play tennis. Even then, I modified poses to help stabilize my knee. I had to find ways to access poses because I WASN'T slender and lithe. And I spent a fair share of time pushing back against the hooey being taught.

In the OLD days, a yoga certification didn't exist. The first class I taught was one I had attended for almost two years. At seventy-five, the instructor decided she'd had enough of teaching yoga and cornered me one day after class. Impressed by my yoga form, she asked if I would like to take over her classes. I thought *what the hell?* At that point, I had secondary teaching certification. How hard could it be to transfer that expertise to the yoga studio?

Not hard, it turns out.

I taught for four years before official certification became a requisite. Even then, it took me almost another year to find a certification program that aligned with my particular style of yoga. The yoga I practice and teach are informed by my injuries. First, fucking up my knee. Later, a broken wrist and clavicle, and recently I shattered my ankle in a fall. I approach yoga with the mindset of an old woman. So imagine my delight when I landed on Viniyoga.

I feel it's safe to say Viniyoga is more closely linked to traditional yoga than some of the hipper, cooler yogas out there. My Viniyoga instructor is so Zen, she finds me amusing.

People come to yoga and think, "Oh, it's a bunch of stretching and whatnot. It's so easy. I don't want to do something easy. It's a waste of my time. I want a real workout. Yoga isn't a real workout." I know because they tell me. To my face. Yes, some yoga is relaxing and easeful. However, even the easy stretching can be a challenge because the majority of folks have short, tight muscles. Almost every client I've met arrived in my class the same way I arrived to that yoga class thirty years ago.

They may slog in, but most rave about how challenging yoga is and how fun I make it.

Everyone thinks yoga teachers are all Zen as fuck and I'm happy to say I know my fair share of pretty amazing yoga teachers. I also know my fair share of yogic assholes. I'm also aware of several well-intentioned yoga teachers who are fine but, fail to offer modifications for clients with specific physical limitations and end up correcting them into problems.

Let's be honest, yoga teachers are humans and therefore aren't immune to the foibles the rest of us struggle to overcome, especially the fucking ego. Make no mistake, yoga teachers can have some serious egos and crazy control issues. Myself included. I mean it takes a little bit of rockstar hubris to perform in front of a class. And as I teacher, I love a captive audience. I try to use my power for good. I'm sure other yoga teachers have good intentions, but you know what they say about the road to hell. It's these kinds of teachers who have ruined yoga for some of us. So much mystical hogwash is offered in some of these studios that your teeth will grind. Once a teacher said, "Twisting rinses out your spinal fluid." I thought I needed emergency dental attention. Eye rolling may not be a yoga pose but I damn sure practice it enough in yoga classes.

Those irritating magazine covers don't help. Let us not forget the supermodels and celebrities claiming to "just love" yoga. I'd like to smack 'em around a bit. Not very yogic, I know.

My yoga brand offers something for every kind of body. In all the years I've practiced and taught yoga, my own form is far from fucking perfect. And you know what? That's okay.

Yoga, taken in its traditional whole is a meta-critical, meta-spiritual concept. Even though I'm keeping the conversation focused on the physical, I'm not dissing the bigger picture.

Believe me, I'm into the groovy yama thing. I practiced Buddhism for almost five years starting in high school. Sure, the bonus was it pissed off my parents, but we also have some crazy rage issues in our family that we attribute to our Aztec Mescalero heritage, and the whole non-violence thing has evened out my jam.

But let me say the hogwash, the hoodoo voodoo, and the bullshit spouted in white, suburban yoga classes, is a gravitational shitstorm so intense, no matter can escape. The quackery I've heard come out of "true" yogis is astounding. When you hear a teacher tell you to feel your anus blossom it ain't no wonder most of us hate yoga.

I have true reverence for the entire philosophy of yoga. The practice aligns with my deep appreciation for the tenets of Buddhism and moves into more modern esoteric practices of The Four Agreements.[2]

Even if you never break on through to the other side, physical yoga is valuable on its own, and saves the lives of my family daily. Yoga and wine, bitches.

---

2   As someone with Aztec ancestry, I'm not sure how I feel about the claims to Toltec wisdom, that said reminding myself to speak with integrity, not to take things personally, to avoid assumptions, and to do your best have kept me out of some scrapes. Not all, but some.

The majority of my clients are only interested in the time they spend on the mat. That isn't a bad thing, however many of the clients I guide, find nuggets of the more profound ideals the physical exercises reveal. I consider that a bonus. And if you don't kill some asshole in the grocery check-out line because you were in my yoga class that day, that's a win.

It's an ongoing conversation with your lifestyle and your body. We forget our bodies serve as our close and intimate companion, rather than just a vehicle to do our bidding. In addition to rebuilding that relationship, I'm trying to keep the conversation lively. The thing is, you have to find the yoga that fits.

You never know what's going to click.

CHAPTER 2

What the fuck IS yoga?

It seems to me a lot of experts are recommending yoga without understanding what yoga is or how it works. What the fuck IS yoga? It's a simple question with a long and complicated answer. A person could devote a lifetime of study to the history, philosophies, and different aspects of yoga, and I know a lot of people who have done that. On the surface, yoga is a way of life. It's a process of changing your perceptions and interactions with the world. It may seem hella intimidating, but how do you eat an elephant? Okay, I wouldn't eat an elephant, but you know what I mean. (One forkful at a time, bitches!)

My answer to this question is: yoga, if we stick with it, it's an opportunity for us to recreate an intimate relationship with our physical bodies. As kids, we inhabited our bodies naturally. You know what I'm talking about; kids delight in wiggling their ears, crossing their eyes, or wrapping their legs around their necks. They don't even think about the how of it. They do it. Practicing yoga reminds us creaky and cranky adults that our shoulders move separately from our arms. Our heads move independently from our shoulders. Our ribs move without regard to our hips. It sounds crazy, but I've had clients discover those small things and have a holy shit moment.

We spend a majority of our lives ignoring or pushing past the messages our body sends us. A lot of us feel the need to do more, go further, or speed faster. Finding a moment to be still and take stock rarely happens. Sometimes we are forced to stop. Typically when we do, it's because we are blindsided by an event, injury or illness. By the time we reach adulthood, we have separated our mental and emotional awareness from our physical body. Think about it; it's ingrained in our culture. No pain, no gain. Cowboy up. Power through it. Suck it up, Buttercup. Those are only a few of the sayings we use to reinforce our belief in the inherent weakness of our bodies. It's systemic and I'm as guilty as anyone of exercising through pain or illness. Ignoring the noises my body is making and pushing through a work out.

I'm not here to transform your life. There are far better resources and far more qualified (and frankly more Zen) yogis out there to guide you along that path if that's your scene. I'm just trying to sum up thousands of years' worth of philosophy, cultural transactions, and modern evolution into manageable bites without boring you into a fucking coma. Hey, wake up!

Yoga, at its most pure, is a philosophic practice of quieting the mind and calming the spirit. Like most religious texts, whose sole purpose, it seems, is to confuse the shit out of us --- the Yoga Sutras, THE book about the eight limbs of yoga philosophy, is told through allegory and metaphor.

For you data nerds (MY PEOPLE):

- Yama: philosophy standards, Golden Rules of integrity;

- Niyamas: elements of self-discipline;

- Asanas: physical poses and movement of yoga;

- Pranayama: manipulation of breath;

- Pratyahara: practice of evaluating ourselves (withdraw our focus from the external to the internal, detaching judgment of others);

- Dharana: act of releasing distractions of the mind (fine-tune one's attention to the space on the mat; breathe, movement, and quality of one's body. *No, not chocolate cake*);

- Dhyana: the gooey ideal; a state of mental stillness while maintaining a connection to breath and body (*meditation, my peeps!*);

- Samadhi: the part of yoga we will carry out of the studio with us; enlightenment, peace, and interconnectedness with all things—if we're lucky.

Hey, I'm happy to leave the mat without the urge to slam the brakes on the jerk who is tailgating me. I like realistic goals and my hubby appreciates the lower insurance rates.

In Sanskrit, yoga literally means *to bind*; to create a union of mind, body, and spirit. Yoga is a process to sharpen the focus of one's thoughts, emotions, and physical existence through the tenets of yoga. Yada, yada, yada.

Somewhere along the line, the yogis of old developed a system of exercises to help us humble mortals build that connection so all three of those things could align in harmony. Insert chanting here. I should mention that I don't fucking chant.[1]

The yoga you typically find at your local gym or recreation center is a physical practice with hoodoo voodoo sprinkled on top. To be accurate, the whole of yoga is a philosophy. For the purpose of this book and my sanity, when I mention *yoga*, I'm referring to the physical practice of it. Traditional practitioners of capital Y yoga grimace when it's discussed purely in these terms. My apologies. (That's much more polite than get over it.) (Just wait until the "Yoga Schmoga" chapter.) Some of those folks are going to light the torches and sharpen the bloody pitchforks.

About 1700 BCE, the Rigveda (*Rig-vay-dah*), one of the four go-to sacred Hindu texts know as the *Samhitas*, mentions yoga. Yeah, you're reading that

---

1   I'd like to go on record that I don't hate chanting. I can't sing. I mean literally, I had surgery on my vocal chords back in the day and it damaged my singing voice. I do enjoy many artists who chant so don't throw that Molotov cocktail just yet.

right. That's nearly two thousand years before the birth of Christ. It's old. And while in its embryonic stage, yoga was strictly a spiritual path; there were a couple of mentions of seated and supine poses to aid in your vision quest. No warriors. No dogs. Nada. Nothing. Naught.

Skip forward a few millennium and bam! The development of yoga poses emerge out of the British colonialization of India. By the 1930s, yoga had become a messy mix of the spiritual and the physical. Sort of a hodgepodge of new fangled ideas with a sprinkle of traditional panoply. We can call it a stew, or should I say molagootal. (Damn it, now I'm hungry.) What we have, is modern transnational physical yoga—a fucking mouthful—so from here on, I'm going to refer to it as MTPY.

People who practice MTPY sometimes reference their type of yoga by lineage. There's a basic (I use the word loosely) family tree connecting the different yoga gurus. Before we discuss the tree, we have to talk about the lingo. You know, the jargon. Ready your pencils.

Hatha (*ha-thah*) in Sanskrit, means *force*. Hatha yoga is the physical form of a pose. In the wide scope of yoga, all physical practice makes up hatha, which includes pose and breath, but Hatha is also the description of a more easeful type of yoga practice. Most studios or gyms include Hatha-type classes. These classifications are a little murky, but hang in there. (I'd like to say it's going to get better, but it's definitely not.)

Ashtanga (*aash-taang-guh*) is the term for the eightfold path of yoga outlined in the Yoga Sutras (THE yoga book). It encompasses the entire mind, body, and spirit.

Asana (*aa-sun-nuh*) Asana is one of those eight paths meaning steady posture, as in, being able to sit for long periods of time. Staying comfortable in your body leads to detachment, known in the eight limbs of yoga as **aparigraha** (*a-par-i-gra-ha*) and relieves suffering. I don't think binging Netflix qualifies, no matter how much or how long I practice.

Ashtanga, no, cool your jets—this is not a typo. This is a second ashtanga. Ashtanga also refers to a more energetic type of yoga. This is all a game of yoga Jenga, so don't wiggle the fucking table.

Vinyasa (*vuh-nyaa-suh*) describes the transition from pose to pose in connection to the breath. In Sanskrit, the word means *arranging in a particular way*. Like ashtanga, vinyasa also describes a type of yoga practice, this one, involving the flowing pattern of positions. Most classes incorporate a vinyasa whether they call it vinyasa or not.

Crystal clear, right? On to the family tree!

I'm going to limit this conversation to colonial and postcolonial physical yoga. Tirumalai Krishnamacharya is widely acknowledged as the father of modern physical yoga, having jumpstarted the physical branch of the eight-limbed path, in the mid 1920s. Krishnamacharya, an ayurvedic healer and scholar hailing from South India in 1888, is considered by yoga peeps to be the source of the poses that make up the bulk of what we practice today. Hang onto this tidbit and keep an open mind, because we're going to veer wildly off of the friggin' track in the "Yoga Schmoga" chapter.

That said, almost everything we practice in MTPY comes from Krishnamacharya's understanding and pursuit of yoga. Krishnamacharya never visited the United States, but many of his students became ambassadors for yoga in the western world.

Probably the most familiar of these teachers is B.K.S. Iyengar. It appears he broke from the philosophical foundation of yoga to focus only on the physical. I like to think he understood a lot of westerners weren't ready for the whole fucking Zen enchilada (or Zenchilada). Iyengar yoga is a hatha variety with a focus on the "perfect pose," categorizing the asanas and the breathing in a specific way that standardized yoga. He was crazy into proper alignment and promoted the use of straps and blocks to cajole (and sometimes force) bodies into what he considered correct position.

Iyengar yoga seems more accessible on the surface because practitioners progressively move from easier poses to more difficult ones. But it's also stricter in terms of "fixing" misalignment. Iyengar yoga is your mother poking your arm with a fucking fork to remind you to keep your elbows off of the table. Well-intentioned, but sometimes too rigid. And yes, I'm judging a little.

K. Pattabhi Jois, another pupil of Krishnamacharya, is linked to ashtanga yoga. Ashtanga yoga is a series of poses that never change in order. It is an energetic practice encouraging powerful and specific breathing rhythms. Think Power Yoga. If you've ever practiced or heard about sun salutations (also known as surya namaskara – *soor-yah nah-mahs-kah-rah*), then you may know the ashtanga style.

Finally, we arrive at Krishnamacharya's son, TKV Desikachar. His philosophy of yoga is dear to my heart because he believed that rather than forcing every person into one perfect, specific alignment, that there was a pose that existed for each person and their particular needs. Desikachar refocused the practice of western yoga on wellness and therapeutic benefit. This is my jam. If you're like me (and almost every other person on the fucking planet) you're coming from injury or illness or a life lived, so this is the yoga for you. Being kind and patient toward yourself can be enough work without worrying about perfect fucking alignment.

Krishnamacharya, check. Iyengar, check. Jois, check. Desikachar, check. All of western yoga can be attributed to these guys whether you've heard of them or not. If you've taken a yoga class, it's likely been one of these styles.

Yoga is the long con.[2] Folks struggle with yoga because it's a patience game. It isn't about instant results. We drove a long and bumpy road to arrive

2   If you aren't familiar with grifters or conman movies, the long con is an elaborate plan that requires a long period of time to get to the payout. Think pyramid schemes without the irritating high school friend who has a great business opportunity.

in our current physical condition. No doubt we made some U-turns. We gained weight. We lost weight. We suffered injury. We got sick. We recovered, or not so much. Some of us had babies. Some of us are just fucking old. All of those things took time, so noticeable changes from yoga, will take time, too.

Here's my basic timeline for getting into a yoga groove. It takes three months to get comfortable on the mat. That means remembering left from right, front from back, and keeping track of those directions while upside down. It takes six more months to figure out exactly what an instructor means when they say "child's pose" or "downward dog" or "forward folding chair." It can take up to a year to discover how to move or adjust your body to receive the full benefits of a pose.

And let me tell you, I have long-practicing clients who come to my class and work through my alignment cues to discover a whole new mojo in their practice.

Well fuck all, Julia, you're not exactly selling it here. I am not going to bullshit you. Even if you decide to commit, you will probably go to yoga class a couple of times a week at best. I'm not judging on this count. Not all of us have the time to practice three hours a week. *Hold up. Three hours a week? Who said anything about three hours a week?* I did. That's my guideline. *Julia, how often should I practice yoga?* Three hours a week. I did tell you yoga is the long con.

Believe me, sometimes it's a tossup between yoga and a glass of wine, but I go because teaching yoga keeps me in wine. A gal has to have priorities.

Even if you get all of those things under control, yoga is still physically, mentally, and emotionally challenging. People make a lot of claims about the benefits of yoga. Some are bullshit and some are science. I like to stick with the science-based ones. No blowing smoke up your ass here. I won't say yoga will help you lose weight because it hasn't helped me lose a single pound. Though some clients swear they've lost weight due to yoga. I won't say yoga will solve your problems because it hasn't solved any of mine. I certainly won't say yoga will help you grow kinder or more patient, though it can happen and that's a big plus. In the philosophy of yoga, this feeling is called purusha (*puh-roo-shah*), the divine spirit or infinite love. It's the transcendence of expectations, judgments, and desires.

There are concrete benefits and I'm living proof:

- Yoga helped me deal with torn MCL and ACL without surgery, so far. (Knock on wood. Throw salt. Run around the house three times naked!)

- Yoga helped me heal from injuries sustained in a serious car accident and my doc said I would have been more critically injured had I not been so strong and flexible.

- I raised three offspring without committing infanticide and I didn't sell them to the gypsies. (Although I may have threatened that on more than one occasion.)
- Yoga helped me recover 95% of full mobility after I shattered my ankle.
- I have the core and upper body strength to wield a sword over my head. (Of course, the Beard has expressly forbidden me from carrying a sword.)

You can ask around, I'm not any more pleasant on the reg, but I haven't stabbed anyone yet. (Make no mistake, I'd like to stab.) Hey, I'm working on it.

Yoga is a fucking glorious thing.

CHAPTER 3

Yoga Nazis Suck

Yoga teachers can have some serious egos. You doubt it? Just look at me.

Yoga teachers do sometimes go to yoga class. I'm one of them. I like to let someone else drive once in a while. And rather than fork over a ton of money to a chi chi[1] yoga studio, I typically go to classes where I pay gym membership. Sometimes that limits the menu selection. There is a teacher who hates me (to be fair, there might be more than one). Shocker, I know. I'm a fucking ray of sunshine. That teacher? She's a yoga Nazi. They exist, both as teachers and as practitioners. There are different categories of yoga Nazis. People can fit into one or all of the different classifications. Alignment Nazis. Timekeeper Nazis. Attendance Nazis. Hippy Dippy Nazis. They run the gamut.

First, let's chat about Timekeeper Nazis. These are yoga instructors who wince when you arrive late or leave early. They get bent out of shape if you

---

1   chi·chi / `SHēSHē, `CHēCHē/ adjective - attempting stylish elegance but achieving only an over elaborate pretentiousness.

don't punch the clock on their schedule. You are fucking with their ability to lead you to Zen. Ha!

Here's the deal . . . while working for other institutions (I'm a former air traffic controller and a former teacher) I was an early morning gym rat. If I didn't work out first thing, it wasn't going to happen. Most days teaching, I was lucky to make it home before I passed out. Never mind exercising in the evening, fuck that. I also happen to be an early morning person by nature. I need my day to start already!

I'd duck out of a class ten minutes early, just before savasana (*sha-va-sa-na*), the final relaxation. I may be a gym rat, but I don't shower at the gym. Cooties, duh. Leaving ten minutes early gave me time to speed home, jump in the shower, and get anywhere I needed to be. Leaving quietly is the polite course to take. If clients tell me they have to leave early, I always recommend bailing before savasana. It's a good time to bolt without disturbing anyone. Even if they don't tell me, I'll give them a cheery wave without judgment.

This bitchy timekeeper ambushed me one day in front of the class with hands on her hips. "You seem to leave class early all of the time."

"I don't seem to, I DO leave early. Every time. I have places I need to be." I don't need my hands on my hips to cop an attitude. Notice I did NOT tell her to go fuck herself. This time. Who says I don't exercise tact?

Most yoga classes are held weekday mornings between eight and nine. This trend caters to clients who don't work. I happen to teach a six a.m. class and a seven-thirty p.m. class during the week. Not everyone is into six a.m. I'm barely into six a.m. Not everyone is into seven p.m. If I weren't teaching the evening class, a large glass of wine sure would be tempting on a Tuesday night. If you come, that's great. If you don't, that's also great.

I know you have lives. Busy lives. Kids, work, laundry . . .whatever. You're not alone. You're welcome in my yoga class any time as long as you're quiet while you're coming or going.

I will give you a nod of greeting if we're in the middle of a hushed part of class to let you know I'm glad to see you. Sometimes I'll out and out wave you into the room. The other day, a couple of young women were peering through the glass during one of my classes. I walked to the door, shooed them right in, and got back to teaching yoga. I want to include everyone.

Just this morning, a new client peeked into the studio thirty minutes late. To be fair, this particular class starts at 6:15 a.m. Yes, in the motherfuck-ing morning. She had overslept and gone to the wrong room. It happens. I brought her in and after class she thanked me. It seems some other teacher had read her the riot act about trespassing on the sanctity of her fucking yoga class. Cuz, we all know that's the epitome of Zen. Sanctity, my ass. My class door is always open. Except during savasana. If the lights are down and the door is closed, stay the fuck out.

And you have to love Attendance Nazis. In the same vein as timekeepers, these are the knobheads who grill you whenever you've been absent from a class for a while. It goes a little like this:

"Hi!" That high-pitched, overenthusiastic tone says they're pissed right off the bat. "Haven't seen YOU in a while." The implication is you had better have a good reason for throwing off their class numbers.

You know what? Fuck 'em. It's none of their goddamn business where you've been or why you haven't been to class. Sure, I'm glad to have full classes. I'm even happier to see regular faces. If you feel like sharing the blazing weekend you spent in Vegas I'll listen, but you are not accountable to me.

Yoga Nazis also hate it when you work their flow slower or faster than they guide. My fitness philosophy is to move smart. Many yoga teachers move too fast. My preference in a yoga flow is moving into a pose and holding for at least three full breaths. Moving at a mindful pace allows a person to be in complete governance of their body. Taking this kind of time ensures control on the mat and offers a body a chance to find its alignment. I've been in classes where teachers are calling out positions in such rapid succession, no one could possibly find the pose safely, let alone get into healthy alignment.

It looks sort of like those promotional air dancers. You know the things that wiggle and flail in front of the cellular stores? And let me tell you, this bitch don't hop.

To be fair, I get a little hot when someone in my class starts throwing down their own thing at a super fast pace. I'll talk more about my reasons in "Slow Your Roll, Bitches." I have been known to have a quiet conversation with a person after class, but I'd never call you out in front of the group. Unless you're locking your elbows. I'm calling that shit out every single time.

The Hippy Dippy Nazi is a practitioner who spouts on and on about the fucking chakras, the auras, your intentions, and aromatic oils. If you are looking for this particular flavor in your yoga, there are studios and specialty classes available. The teachers in these classes sound a little like this: [in a breathy voice] *Close your eyes. Imagine the* [insert number here] *chakra. The color of this chakra is blah. The emotional issues represented by this chakra are* [insert some voodoo bullshit here]. *This chakra is enhanced, transformed, and energized by this aromatic oil. Go deep into your mind and listen to your higher self for the intention you should be focusing on in this practice.*

Stop fucking yapping already! And don't rub my hair with that goddamn oil. In a gym, recreation center, or health club, unless the class is specifically designed to address these topics, it's a sneak attack. Don't get me wrong, I respect my higher self though I consider it more of a listening-to-your-intuition thing. And I love me some aromatic oils. I'm all about the eucalyptus oil in the shower (or in the sauna if I had one . . . hey hubby?) when I have a cold. I dig me some lavender oil on the pillow at night, and I'm all about the basil/tea tree oil cleaner in the kitchen.

But to have to listen to the color of the chakra and which oil transforms what energy in a yoga class causes me more rage than any amount of breathing can ease. Also, don't drip shit on me. Seriously, no yoga teacher should rub any kind of substance on you without prior understanding and clear consent. Actually, that's just a good general life rule. Am I right? I have clients with all sorts of allergies and sensitivities. I don't need a fucking lawsuit.

A friend of mine shared her aversion to yoga. In her mid-twenties, she attended a certain brand of hot yoga. It happened to be her first yoga class ever. (I would never recommend hot yoga to a beginner. Hot yoga is a vigorous practice in the Ashtanga model performed to precise and exacting standards in a room heated to one-hundred-and-four degrees Fahrenheit, bleh.) Overheating, my friend stopped to take a drink from her water bottle and received a prompt and loud rebuke from the instructor in front of the entire group. It wasn't the prescribed point in the practice for her to drink the water. She never went to another yoga class again. She hasn't even been to mine. She was scarred by a fucking Yoga Nazi.

Clients bitch to me about the Drill Sergeant Nazi. Music so loud you can barely concentrate on your mat. These Nazis bark out orders at the top of their lungs and spew things like, "Ignore your body! Demand the pose from your mind! Push down your discomfort! Disconnect your brain!" Even in the context of yoga equaling physical practice for this book that, my friends, is exactly the opposite of fucking yoga.

And then there is the Orator Nazi. Oh, for the love of Pete! These are the yoga wankers who talk and talk and talk and talk. They lecture about the origins of the pose (usually bullshit, btw). They discuss the intent of the practice with minutia. Worse, they tell some sort of inspirational story, which is really an ego-fest on how illuminated they are. Words, words, words, words. Hell on toast and shut the fuck up!

Sure, I talk poses and offer verbal cues. I'll even give the names of poses, mostly in English, but I love the Sanskrit. It's mouth porn. I remind clients of healthy alignment. Soften your elbows, lift and spread your toes, keep breathing. Those are normal in a yoga class. Once everyone has the flow of the practice anchored in their mind, I shut the fuck up. Give people a chance to get into their space. Find the gooey center of the Zen. Go ahead and snort, but I'll sell you on the goo eventually.

Not only do these kinds of classes give yoga a terrible rep, but they also create a horrible misunderstanding of what yoga can be. They remove any hint of the original intentions. Yes, I'm fucking judging. A yoga practice should serve the practitioners. As a yoga rockstar, I am in the studio to help you find your best practice. I've said it before, and I'll likely say it again. Yoga is a tool to establish a connection between your body and your mind. I may not address the tenets of yoga as a whole directly, but I am mindful of them in every practice.

I dig the fact that in most of western society, a workout is expected to be a challenge. Hey, I was a runner, more of a plodder. I'm a cycle instructor. If cycle class isn't a recipe for a heart attack or a hot flash, or hurling, I don't know what is. A part of me loves the tough work while an equal part of me despises it. Have I mentioned I'm the worst fitness instructor ever? I'm not a cheerful gym person. I have trouble with the "Aren't we having so much fun?" line because even though I'm teaching, I'm not having fun. If I yell, "Whoo!" it translates into "Holy Fuck! This sucks!" Talk to me after a shower and a double espresso or depending on the time of day, a glass of wine. That's when I love working out.

Yoga ain't for sissies. Practiced with a mindful focus and with well-planned thought, yoga can be a challenge on multiple levels. That's its fucking purpose. Effective instructors can transmit this philosophy without overpowering the general audience with the esoteric language of the Sutras, which many of them don't actually understand. I can guide mindfulness and the three-part breath without losing my average, non-hippy segment. And I can encourage the grace and kindness I preach to clients without cheating them out of a physically demanding experience. No yelling required. Okay, I am loud, but for the most part I get down to business.

Yoga, the whole of yoga, the fucking grande burrito of it all, is about embracing and connecting. Embracing and connecting with your current physical, mental, and emotional states. Embracing and connecting with a community of people working toward similar goals. Embracing and connecting with the awkwardness and aches and kinks and crackles we all deal with on a daily fucking basis.

Dharana (*dah-rah-nah*) is the act of dealing with the distractions of the mind. And as we embrace and connect with our body in a pose, we are constantly flitting from one thought to another. If we can move past the different stages of noise and settle our focus on inhabiting our bodies, we arrive at Dharana, the act of effortless engagement. If you are dealing with Yoga Nazis, it's hard not to punch someone, but hey, I'm working on it.

CHAPTER 4

Yoga Ain't for Sissies

Well, that doesn't sound very yoga-ish. Where is all of your welcoming Zen hodgepodge? Who's the Yoga Nazi now, Julia?

Hold up. I'm going to tell you a story. You know, if you roll your eyes they can stick like that. I told you that in my previous life I was a gym rat. There's a distinction between gyms and health clubs even though the terms are often interchangeable. In my experience, gyms are typically steel-sided, commercial buildings in industrial parks. Gyms have three or four sets of free weights, every kind of weight bench imaginable, and step frames. Space is cavernous. Ain't no one going to bump elbows while they're on the incline bench. They may have a handful of weight machines, mostly so they have somewhere to place chin up bars, and in whatever space may be left, they might put in a few treadmills, bikes, and perhaps an elliptical machine or two. They might have a few televisions. And you damn well better bring your own towel.

Again, in my experience, gym folk are cheerful without being too chatty, and they have serious respect for gym etiquette. No one is going to ask you how your weekend was. They don't really care. They'll spot you and come save you if you fuck up with the barbell, but it's not a social hour. You'll probably find a locker room and perhaps a steam room that is out of service more often than not. Chic workout clothes are rarely on display and I've never had someone try to pick me up in a gym. Ever. We're all there to work out. Grrrrrrrr (everybody flex like Ahhnold).

Health clubs might have one set of free weights, two if you're lucky, crammed into a corner. They have every weight machine known in the free world and all manner of cardio machines, each with their own personal television screen along with an entire wall of televisions. They hand out fluffy towels in multiple sizes at the desk and always smile cheerfully no matter how much you growl at them. Health clubs often have pools and a hot tub. Typically, the rules are posted on the walls, along with restrictions on machines, because sometimes particular classes are scheduled to use them. The selection of runway workout gear is blinding.

Health club folks run the gamut. There are cheerful, chatty folk, and snooty folk. To be fair, the snooty folk might just be miserable, but they enjoy radiating the misery, infecting everyone else in the joint. They typically don't know workout etiquette, and they get snippy when you explain they've jumped your round. The cheerful chatters have coffee, and they move in packs while talking about every detail of their lives: the weather, or whatever, while leaning on the equipment. They also love to draw other people into chats whenever they're alone. And if they see you regularly, they keep track of when you're gone.

"Hey, you must've been taking it easy last week."

"What? You decided to sleep in?"

Never mind, you probably had the fucking flu, or your kid had the flu or it's just none of their goddamned business. Okay, I am breathing.

I worked out at a local gym for many years. The building opened at four-thirty a.m. for crazy people like me, along with a handful of morning regulars whose faces grew familiar over time. After a couple of years, we started nodding at each other. There was a gaggle of guys who worked out together. Three or four BIG guys. Linebacker guys. Not a one of them was shorter than six-foot-two, and the smallest might have weighed two-forty. They were generally polite and kept conversation at the lowest decibel. I do know one of them was nicknamed Big Jim possibly to distinguish him from little Jim. Not making that up. These guys loved throwing the massive weights around. If they used the free weights, they were no less than fifty pounds. These guys were huge.

I'd go in before dawn, return their nods, and go work with three pounds, five pounds, maybe on a crazy day, ten pounds. If I worked with the barbell, I often used a light or no weight. I have a tendency to turn into Helga the Power Lifter if I use heavy weights. Even at my ideal size, it's hard to find long sleeves that fit my upper arms. Fuck that. As a yoga instructor, I know how to use light weights to maximum benefit, and I'm always thinking about being in control of my body weight. It took about three years before we moved past the nods and started saying, "Morning." Another entire year went by before the body builder types started with the snorts and elbows to each other over my weight routines.

These guys threw, and I mean threw one-hundred-pound free weights around using momentum to get their curls complete. They had enormous, but short muscles. Enormous muscles are HEAVY muscles. I knew these guys had zero control over their own body weight. Their teasing was good-natured. I didn't worried about it. After all, I was one of them, a gym rat. I laughed them off for a while until one day I decided to put these knuckleheads to the test.

"All right, guys, I'm going to challenge you. Three tests and if I beat you, you're gonna knock it off with the *'should we get you a pink set of weights'* routine."

With grins and a lot of nudging, they agreed. They could out-muscle me.

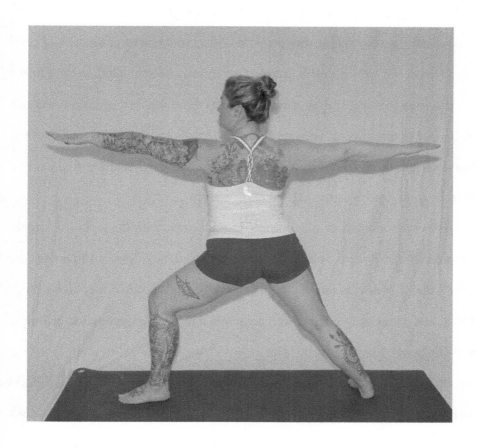

Test one entailed standing with feet about hip width and holding out a set of free weights in a T-position with a slight bend in the elbows, for sixty seconds. This is virabhadrasana II arm position (warrior two). Zero momentum; you must manage the posture with absolute control. I went first to demonstrate with my three-pound dumbbells. Cake and pie. A piece of cake, a slice of pie. (Thank you, Dean Koontz, for one of my favorite sayings.) Big Jim grabbed his sixty-pound weights (I recommended they choose the lightest weight they worked with. I'm not a total bitch) and tried to lift them into position. He strained, grunted, and struggled. It took him a good minute or two, but he managed to get them up. Ten or fifteen seconds in he lost it, and his arms came flopping down. It's one thing to lift a big, heavy weight with a gathering of momentum. It's another thing to lift it and hold it up as dead weight with no extra energy.

Test two consisted of one complete chest press with heels on the bench, shoulder blades spread open, back pressed completely down so that the core engaged and your ribs tuck in. Note: this is not the accepted form for a Huge Dude bench press. It is, however, a more total body engagement technique and it's better for your back. This position requires absolute control of the weight and often means you must slow down your movements. A lot of folks arch their backs up and push out with their rectus abdominis (the six-pack muscle) while pressing their feet on the floor, especially when the weight is heavy. (Ladies, a little hint. Any muscle you bulge out while exercising is going to get bigger in that direction. (I don't know many women who are thrilled if their belly is bulkier.) One of the other guys gave it a shot and yes, he was able to work the bar up, but not control it on the way down.

Test three was my favorite: one complete sit-up on the decline bench from lowest position to highest position without an arm swing or any other push of momentum. By this time, the manly muscle crew, as I'm now calling them, were laughing, poking at each other. Failure imminent, they humored me and gave it a go.

By this time, they knew they would fail. Ginormous upper bodies weigh A LOT. They couldn't even get their backs off of the bench.

In the end, their workout routines remained unchanged, however, they'd bow and wink at me when I came into the gym. Meh. I would've loved to get those guys hooked on yoga, but it would've meant a significant paradigm shift in their exercise routine.

Yoga ain't for sissies.

Remember when I said some people think, "Oh, it's nothing but stretching and whatnot?" Once folks get into a healthy alignment, they discover how friggin' heavy their arms, their head, and their legs can be. It's awesome! (Yes, I did singsong that a little.)

However, this is where a yoga practice can go off of the rails. Many yoga classes are designed for people who crave a punishing workout, and healthy alignment disappears.

Yoga takes time and patience. Recall the timeline. Three to six months to get the hang of it. In an effective class, you'll discover all the ways your body is designed to move, many of them long forgotten. Once you learn how your body moves, you have to work past muscle memory and habit. This is true in different ways for both the young and those of us who are older.

Young women tend to hyperextend because they are hyper flexible and tend to have less muscle strength. They hang out on their locked joints, particularly the hips. Terrible for posture. Your mother is right, stop slouching.

Older women tend to slouch for different reasons, especially if they're large breasted. (Everyone just sat up straight. You know you did.) Most people slouch because our lives are designed to reinforce it. The sofas we sit on, the computers we work on, the sink, the stove, the fridge, the car—all forward work.

If you're a runner or a cyclist, you might have chronic lower backache. Running and cycling are primarily forward work mainly using quadriceps and hamstrings. Anecdotally, nine times out of ten, people are not effectively stretching to compensate. Don't deny it. I've already called you out on it. Even if I demand a blood oath that you'll spend at least ten minutes some time during the day to stretch, you won't. I don't judge . . . okay, bullshit, in this case I am judging, but only because I know you'll pay for it in the long term.

And don't give me that "You can overstretch" bullshit. I know you can overstretch, but ten to fifteen minutes of good stretching post cycle or circuit class is not going to cause harm. Remember, yoga isn't just about stretching. It's stretch *and* strength. Longer muscles help prevent other injuries. Stronger core muscles and leaner strength can improve balance, which leads to flexibility, thus, preventing injuries. Stretching strong muscles can reduce imbalance from repetitive work. Working on the computer. Hunching over your mobile. Washing dishes. (Does cleaning the kitchen ever fucking end?) Hiking a toddler on your hip. That's why it's important to vary your exercise routine. More balanced strength overall lessens push and pull from overly strong muscles, reducing misalignment and what? Preventing fucking injuries.

You pickin' up what I'm throwing down?

Longevity, people. That's the name of the game. Active, healthy, and flexible into your fifties, sixties, and beyond. Haven't you heard the eighties are the new forties?

Men often struggle with this concept more than women because biologically, men have more powerful upper body structure. Women typically have heavier lower body strength. Over the course of evolution, our bodies developed to serve us more successfully, thus, ensuring our survival. It makes no difference. Starting a yoga practice is a challenge one way or another for everyone. I do appreciate men in yoga class because they make noise. They grunt. They groan. They oomph. Not because they're whiners, but because they're more comfortable acknowledging hard work. Women tend to suffer in silence. The clown car should put a cork in it.

Are you sick of hearing it yet? Yoga ain't for sissies. (Repetition is a key characteristic of effective communication.) It's both physically and mentally challenging and demands a commitment to process, a long-term process. But trust me, you can do it. And when someone air quotes the fact that "you're doing yoga" because they think it's all gooey, give them a serene smile and walk away while throwing them two big old birds.

Ahimsa is the practice of non-violence. I'm working on it.

CHAPTER 5

Don't Fucking Touch Me

Remember when I said yoga helped me heal my ankle? A few years ago, in the course of saving a neighbor's toddler from a passing car, I slipped on the ice. Shattered my ankle.

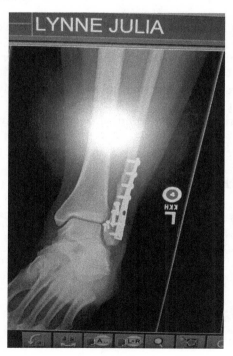

Okay, I actually stepped off my front porch while taking the damn trash out and slipped. I did break my ankle. Coincidentally, it was early before my Saturday yoga classes. I didn't have my phone. The dogs and my hubby (with ear plugs) were asleep at the opposite end of the house. The offspring slept in the friggin' basement. After a robust and colorful round of swearing, I crawled from the driveway back into the house and hollered for help. You ever feel like your life is a fucking sitcom? Ten screws and a five-inch rod later, I was fixed. Mostly.

The fall happened in February. I couldn't bear weight until May, and then I wore a stylish and sleek contraption affectionately known as 'Das Boot.' If you've haven't been there; first, you lay in bed a lot. Eventually, you move around on a scooter, ideally one with brakes. Trust me, brakes are a must. After that, you use crutches and then move to a cane. My hubby denied me a Gandalf staff on the grounds I might be tempted to swing it at deserving assholes at the grocery store. Resist the urge to burn the boot. I recommend keeping it, the crutches, and the cane for at least a year in the case of recurring surgery. It might be wash, rinse, and repeat. I learned that the hard way. It's a barrel of fun, let me tell you.

Returning to yoga was a delicate process. Interesting fact: bones flex. Seriously. In the context of the kinetics of your body, your bones have a little bit of room to give and flow to your movement. Steel rods screwed to the bones don't fucking flex. Not only does this cause issues up the chain in your typical day-to-day operation, it also thrashes a fucking yoga practice. Your alignment in a particular asana is, to put it technically, whacked as fuck. Yes, that is a technical yoga term.

I returned to teaching yoga pretty quickly after gaining my feet—one of them at any rate. Over time and in strict accordance with my physical therapist, I got back on the mat with intent. My goal? Earn back one hundred percent of my dorsiflexion. My dorsi-what? Your foot moves in multiple directions pivoting around the ankle. Y'all just picked up your foot and rolled your ankles around, didn't you? Goddamn the body is amazing, isn't it? When you point your toes, it's plantar flexion, and when you flex your foot toward your shin, it's dorsiflexion.

Another true story, no, really true this time— I hate to be touched. I spent eleven years in the secondary classroom grades six through twelve. Sixth graders like to hug. Apparently those elementary teachers are all big fuzzy teddy bears. Me? I'm more of a Grizzly. It became a game to them. Who could ambush Ms. Lynne with a hug and avoid being clotheslined?

For all of the years I've practiced and taught yoga, my own practice is far from fucking perfect. I gushed a bit about TKV Desikachar. The primary tenet of his philosophy was "teach to the individual." I often have as many as twenty-five people in a class. Not one of us looks or moves like the other. There is no such thing as the perfect pose. If a yoga instructor doesn't know you're recovering from an injury; if you've had surgery; if you are knock-kneed; or cross-eyed—okay, that one might be a given, they can cause damage. This is worth repeating . . . unless a yoga teacher is an accredited yoga therapist or a licensed physical therapist who has spent quality time getting to know you and your physical history, they can adjust you right into a fucking injury.

Many fitness instructors hate the sight of me because I participate in the activity in a manner that is kind to my body. It doesn't mean I'm not working hard. I'm working smart. And little-known fact: many yoga teachers are dumbass control freaks. Even if a teacher is suggesting something that flies in the face of my philosophy, I can generally find a way to work with the practice.

Oh, they can talk auras and chakras and the sutras and aromatic oils out the wazoo. They can speak in dulcet, calming tones, but trust me; some of them aren't walking the walk. I've experienced fuckwit teachers who yank, tug, push, and basically force clients into their idea of "perfect pose" without any consideration for the client.

Remember, yoga teachers can have massive egos (me too). Yoga Nazis, anyone?

These kinds of teachers are quick to pounce on perceived misalignment and form. If an instructor is going around correcting alignment, I politely inform them that I prefer not to be corrected. Don't roll your eyes, I do! The first time, maybe even the second time. The final time I firmly and quietly say, "Don't fucking touch me." The last yoga teacher I pissed off tried to get me into better alignment during an asana called warrior two (virabhadrasana II). She didn't ask. She aggressively pulled my knee into what she thought was perfect alignment. After a brief moment of surprise, I informed her to fuck off as the five-inch rod in my ankle prevented my knee from being in the alignment she wanted. Mind you, I'd already been added to her "I hate this client" list because I scooted out of class before savasana. I'm telling you, control freaks.

This kind of correction happens more often than I like. I recently bumped into a regular client at the grocery store (small towns), and she explained she was taking a couple of weeks off because her wrists were killing her. She had attended another class where the instructor corrected her hand placement into perfect ninety-degree alignment over her wrists during tabletop (I call it hands and knees).

"Why didn't you just ignore her?" I asked, thinking of all of the times I've told my clients not to allow dumbass instructors to adjust them into a position they know doesn't work for their bodies.

She shrugged. "It was like I was back in first grade and the teacher scolded me, and I just did it."

After a shattered wrist and carpal tunnel surgery (I swear I'm not a klutz), I discovered a more easeful placement of the hands further out in front of my shoulders. I cue, "Move your hands a half to a full palm's length in front of your shoulders." After thirty years of yoga, it changed my fucking life. As it was an epiphany, I now make it part of my yoga gospel to others. I want you to practice yoga until you're ninety. Hell, past ninety if you have it in you.

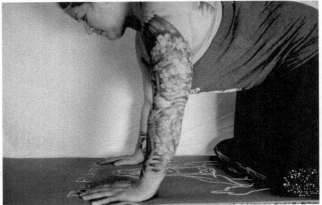

Avoid this.

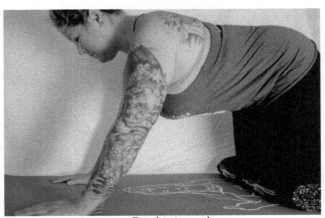

Do this instead.

I do adjust alignment in my classes. Not to get you further into a pose. Nine times out of ten, I'll ask a client to ease up on a pose. Yoga isn't a competitive sport. Sure, it's fine to peek out the corner of your eye to see what fucking foot is where and which fucking direction we're facing but no one's yoga looks the same as another's. It must be clear, your yoga won't look like mine, and even after thirty years, my yoga doesn't look like my yoga teacher's. Remember, body type, physical history, and fitness levels (both out of fit and being super fit) can change how you move.

Invariably, I see clients moving too far into poses. Over stretching, over-reaching, going too deep. Pain is bad. Pain is your body's way of saying, "Hey, damage here, bitch! We're experiencing damage!" Discomfort is a different animal. There is such a thing as over stretching. Believe me, a ligament strain or muscle tear is so much fucking worse than a clean bone break. Recovery from soft tissue damage is long and painful. And often, I see clients stretching MORE because they think it's a tight muscle thing.

There's this thing called yoga butt. It's a terrible pain at the base of your sit bones and feels like tight hamstrings. Really, it's a strain, either of the Sacrotuberous ligament or of the fascia connecting the hamstring to the sit bones. The inclination is continued stretching, but you can be causing more fucking strain of the area.

A cycling instructor I know uses the term "comfortably uncomfortable." I like that idea. Yoga is about becoming familiar with the unfamiliar. Getting to know an old friend. Grace and kindness, people.

There is strong and healthy alignment as opposed to "perfect" alignment and it's different for every body. I tell my clients every single class that yoga isn't about how close you can get your toes to your nose. It's about discovering the length of your leg from hip to heel. There's a difference between a person's face in pain and a person's face as they discover a new and interesting way their body moves. A sound usually escapes with the latter. It's sort of an Oooohhhh sound. I don't make this shit up. It happens every fucking time.

I often see people struggle to get into a pose when they clearly need some help or a different way to approach it. And you can hang at the very back of my class; I'll still see you. Hello! I was a middle school teacher. I can spot injuries, or imbalances because your body can't lie. The path you've taken in life must inform a better fucking way to do yoga. A good instructor is there to help you find your individual approach.

Case in point: I have a hubby and wife who are more recent regulars. In the last vinyasa class, we worked through a plank pose called kumbhakasana (*koom-bah-kah-sah-nah*). After class, she asked me about some calf stretches and mentioned she had injured her calf. She drew up her pant leg to show me. That fucker was eggplant purple from knee to ankle. That wasn't just injured. That fucker was probably torn.

"What should I be doing to stretch this out?" She asked. "I was struggling in plank."

"Uh, no fucking wonder," I said. "First, that would have been a really good thing to mention before class. Second, get thee to a doctor and have that shit examined. Third, not a goddamn thing for at least six weeks," I said.

"I TOLD you!" Her hubby said. "I told her."

"But it's been a week," she argued.

"It's been THREE DAYS!" Hubby shouted. "And you went snowboarding yesterday."

I put my hands up. "Normally, I'd tell your hubby to leave you be, but in this case, I'm siding with him. You must rest your calf until there is zero discoloration. I'm not talking greenish or yellow. I'm talking completely normal. No plank, unless you are modifying on your knees. Zero downward facing dog. Maybe some light calve raises and VERY EASY stretching, but nothing more."

"NOTHING?!" She squawked.

"Nothing," I said.

"Nothing," her hubby repeated firmly.

"And if you come to yoga, you best believe I'll be watching you to ensure you are not pushing," I said. I shot her the I'm-watching-you gesture.

This is exactly the mindset that yoga, my yoga, helps break. I may not offer the Yamas or Niyamas in general, but I guide clients toward svadhyaya (*svahd-yah-yah*), or more specifically, self-study, to know oneself. Niyamas are the physical observances of the eight limbs. The more we practice yoga, the more we exist within our bodies with awareness. This is the exact opposite of cowboy up. No one knows your body better than you do. Remember, pain is bad. Pain is our warning system. Never hesitate to talk to an instructor and inform them, confidently, of your limitations or injuries. I tell people every single class, if I know you're recovering from an injury or have some hindrance I can make you infinitely more comfortable in a pose. It never fails. I ease someone into a better position and the light goes on. "Oh my! That's so much better!"

You know it, bitches!

CHAPTER 6

Yoga Isn't An Express Ticket To Hell

I've got nothing against religion. Okay, I have a few of things against religion; no objections related to the spiritual charity and altruism preached, but mostly related to assholes. I'm pretty sure it's a friggin' rule or law in all religions. Don't be an asshole. It's pretty good life advice too. Thanks to my dear friend, Curtis for the boil down. I run into holy rollers all of the time. Yoga will corrupt your soul. That ink on your body is just an invitation to the demon. Swearing is a sin and will bar you from entering the gates. You're going to be eternally damned. Puh-leez. If those are the benchmarks, I've already dropped that fucking basket.

A friend of mine was ambushed by her minister (yes, I'm friends with a Christian, duh. Clearly, she's not an asshole) after someone tattled that she had started going to yoga class. The minister lectured her in a passionate and horrifying way on the dangers to her soul. The very depths of hell would open with fire and brimstone to swallow her yoga mat. She would bring the coming of the plagues, especially feet fungus of those pagan hippies in her class, to all of humanity. Horns would sprout from her head lest she give up any attempt of headstands. Okay, we'll cover feet issues in "Who Let the Dogs Out," but the rest is bullshit.

More recently, some douchebag mega-church guy says Hinduism is demonic. Uh, no. There's so much to unpack there, I just can't. More to the point, MTPY isn't intrinsically a part of Hinduism. Because this is a yoga book, I'm going to ignore the larger argument of cultural appropriation in terms of Christmas being celebrated on the pagan holiday of Yule or Halloween being a variant of the pagan holiday Samhain or Easter as the Christian celebration of the resurrection is literally Eostre, the Saxon/German god of dawn and spring and uh, rebirth. Until later that is.

If you haven't noticed, we've arrived at one of my bête noirs. I'm keeping the list related to yoga, sheesh. Yoga isn't a fucking religion. It's an activity designed to create a calmer mind, a more peaceful emotional state, and a better understanding of who you are. Self-awareness. This is covered in part, by the Yamas and Niyamas. The Yamas address the moral aspects of our behavior, non-violence, truthfulness, non-stealing, non-possessiveness, and sexual moderation. The Niyamas cover our personal behavior, purity, contentment, discipline, devotion, and self-study. I got no problem with truthfulness. It's the non-violence that trips me up every fucking time, but I'm working on it.

Yoga can be practiced within any religion. While yoga taken in its traditional whole is a meta-critical, meta-spiritual concept that can include physical practice, you're not going to hell. And even though I'm keeping the conversation focused on the physical, I'm not dissing the bigger picture. Believe me, I'm into the groovy, niyama thing, but not everyone is. And most of the things I hear from most yoga instructors has little basis in actual yoga philosophy.

My recipe for yoga is more of a Cajun boil. Tie on that bib, pour on the Beaujolais, and let's dig in with our hands. Yoga for the 99%, yah know? If I'm going to hell, at least I know there will be a party.

Even talking strictly physical practice, I can hide a little Zen in there with the best of 'em. I used to scold my middle school students with one word. Elevate. Frankly, we could all use a little fucking elevation. Elevate means to raise your mind out of the gutter and remember the Golden Rule. Treat others not how you are treated, but how you would like to be treated. Okay, I stole it. Not only am I paraphrasing good ol' Gandhi, but MOST of the major religions would agree. I would tell those students, "Remember to elevate your thoughts because your thoughts become words and words become your actions."

I think it's a pretty good life philosophy. While it may be spiritual, it is not religion.

A lot of my clients find a satisfaction in yoga they can't quantify. Call it Zenning out, call it mindfulness, or call it 'Holy shitballs, my brain was quiet for five entire minutes." Many of them have taken the next step and tried an actual meditation class. At the least, you might find the presence of mind to be calmer and kinder when faced with the fucking bastards in your world. If that isn't enough, you can lower your blood pressure, find relief to minor aches or fatigue, or notch down your stress and irritation. It's a win-win.

Savasana (*sha-va-sa-na*) is final relaxation and it's the cherry on top of any yoga practice. First, you have to get over the translation; sava in Sanskrit means corpse. Sava + asansa equals corpse pose. Yeah, it's because you lie like a dead body. Savasana is expected to be the final pose in any solid yoga practice. I'll admit if I'm practicing on the road by my lonesome, I take a short, seated meditation.

Savasana is traditionally somewhere around ten to fifteen minutes. Some yoga sources say a minute for every minute of practice. Personally, I check the vibe of the class. If they're going with the yoga flow, I'll run a full ten-minute savasana. In a beginning class, I often keep it down to six minutes. Resting silently on the floor with your eyes closed (I usually play some kind of peaceful music) with a group of people you don't know can be nerve-wracking. Sometimes your brain doesn't know how to settle down. How do I know everyone has their eyes closed? Did I just nod off? If I did, did I snore? Did I turn the coffee machine off? Oh shit, I hope my hubby, kid, partner, parent remembered to [fill in the blank] ? Relax! I said RELAX! I just know someone is watching me. Did that guy just fart?

I'd be remiss if I didn't mention the super sexy side of yoga. Someone is going to fart and someone is going to snore. Go ahead and giggle, then let's move on.

Savasana is meant to be a quiet, meditative state. I talk a class down using a blend of shitali karana (*shee-tah-lee kar-ah-nuh*) (ascending breath) and yoga nidra (union/aware sleep). These methods allow folks to focus on something other than the noise in their brain. Settling into savasana in my class takes a minute or two. We remain in Savasana for up to seven minutes before I talk them back out of it. In a beginning class, we may lie for three to five minutes, or I may have people count their breaths. It all depends on the crowd. This is the seed of mindful quiet that can find its way into the rest of your yoga practice the more you do it.

I have a client who travels for a living. She swears by her fifteen-minute savasana. "I just pretend I hear your voice in my head and I run through savasana. I can sleep anywhere. Doesn't matter how crappy the hotel is."

Regular practice of yoga also opens a recognition of the physical quality of the body you may have ignored. A closer understanding of the way your body works and feels can help with all sorts of issues. Remember svadhyaya? You know, self-studying? Noticing aches and pains can lead to better alignment and posture. Your physical form is your closest, most intimate friend. You spend a good majority of your life ignoring it, punishing it, and abusing it. We wouldn't treat a neighbor with the same negativity with which we treat our own bodies. If a neighbor were ill, we wouldn't say, "Suck it up and get your ass moving, bitch." We'd recommend rest, hot tea, or maybe make soup. We would NOT say of an injured neighbor, "Oh that bad neighbor is such a pain in the ass." We'd offer to shovel their walk or show up on their porch with a meal. Okay, not in my neighborhood because I'm me, but you get the gist.

Last time I checked this was the man from Galilee's jam. Grace and kindness. I recall a tenet about showing hospitality to strangers and entertaining angels unaware. I know there are all manner of fairy tales and folk stories about failing to be kind to those less fortunate than yourself and getting your ass cursed. So we're round to the notion that while yoga ain't a fucking religion, it's certainly not the descent into hell fire some asshole is preaching.

Even if you don't find a reserve of good vibrations to share, over time you grow more comfortable in your skin. You'll spend a lot of time growing an awareness of what feels better. Whenever I'm out of factory settings, I know I need to take some action. It might be a visit to the doc or simply getting more sleep, but I can always tell when shit isn't copacetic. You'll get into the habit of treating your body better when it needs it.

Fucking yoga, baby.

I remind clients if they blow out their knee, it may be weakened, but it's not BAD—like bad dog! Yoga is a strategy to remember our body serves us as best it can and sometimes, we treat it very shabbily. Grace and kindness are often the hardest to offer ourselves. So while absolutely not a religion, yoga can bring you back to a place where you recognize yourself and help put some perspective on what's happening around you. If we learn patience for ourselves, we can develop patience for other people that are not us.

I will nurture santosha (that's contentment) in line at the grocery checkout. I will, goddamn it.

CHAPTER 7

I AM Breathing, Bitch

I've learned from my time on the mat a lot of people hate to fucking breathe. I'm talking, *loathe*. It's not that they don't breathe, rather, it's the concentration on the breath that causes frustration, stress, and downright hostility. We spend ninety percent of our time breathing intuitively. It's automatic. Drawing focus to automatic functions creates glitches in the system. Have you blinked your eyes recently? We rarely think about blinking our eyes unless that one fucking particulate gets in and you can't for the life of it get it out. And sure as shit, you just blinked. It's like that. I have two friends whom I still haven't been able to get into my yoga class because they don't want to breathe. They don't even want to hear about breathing. Did you read about that woman in Texas bickering with her husband? She shot him. I'm pretty sure he said, "It's not a big deal. Just take a deep breath, honey." Oh relax, he's still alive. My point is, concentrating on breathing is a legitimate fucking obstacle.

Many people associate deep breathing with meditation, and that can be a wrong way path down a one-way road. I meditate. I don't sit fucking still and breathe meditate. I don't make the time. Frankly, I struggle with the sitting still thing. I've got laundry to do. I've got dust bunnies to ignore. I've got books to write and a hundred other things I choose to devote time over sitting still and breathing. I do however breathe. Daily. Approximately twenty thousand breaths.

No I didn't fucking count. I'm figuring I breathe deeper than the average person and the average breath count is somewhere around twenty-five to thirty thousand a day. To be fair, I teach a lot of fitness classes and practice yoga breathing. That's a lot of ins and outs to be cheating yourself of full oxygen. And yes, sometimes in a fitness class I take a little extra time to explain exercises because I'm trying to breathe, goddamn it.

In the broader eight-limbed path of yoga, one of the focuses is the Pranayama. Prana is considered energy: nutrition, water, and breath. Ayama means expansion or mastery. In this case, mastery over Prana. Pranayama is most commonly discussed in terms of breathing. But as part of the eight-limbed path, it includes the rest. Of course, eating healthy provides good energy. No, Golden Oreos aren't a good source of energy. Yes, they are yummy. YES, they fucking ARE. But no, they're not nutritious. Just saying. Hydration (as in water, not wine), keeps us lubricated and balanced. Every cell in our body needs it. All right, sometimes every cell in our body calls out for wine too. However, the ruler, the king, the mostest of Prana, is breath.

There is an allegory about breath that one of my teachers told me. One afternoon, the forces of Prana were hanging out in the shade of a tree discussing their importance. I don't know why, they just fucking were. Okay? Food puffed its chest and said, "I'm the most critical, bitches. Just watch, without me there is nothing." But a body can last several days without food. Nutrition returned bent out of shape. So Water strutted next. "I must be the most important. Nothing can last without me." But a body can survive many days without water. So Water returned also acting like somebody pissed in the pool. They each looked at Breath expectantly. "Well?" They demanded. Breath smiled, said nothing, and left. They quickly called Breath back, because when Breath leaves, life fucking ends. It's done, over, finito.

When you hear pranayama in a yoga class, we're usually only talking breath. Wait? Breathing? Seriously, it's just in and out, isn't it? If any of you have delivered a baby or been present during delivery or seen a portrayal of a delivery you know of what I speak. First thing in a crisis or stressful situation, people say, "Breathe." Sure, you may want to brain them with whatever object is handy, but it's not for fucking nothing. There are studies from all over the medical field proving the benefits of just a few minutes of deep breathing every day.

Think about maintaining a deep breathing rhythm for an entire hour.

The basis for all yoga breathing is called the Dirga (*deer-gah*), the three-part breath that focuses on belly, diaphragm, and chest (there is also an entirely different breathing thing that involves retention and suspension, but that's a completely different jam.) The pattern of breathing changes depending on the desired results. I shit you not. In viniyoga, the general rhythm of breathing starts with the expansion of the chest and progresses down through the ribcage and finally into the abdomen. Pretty intuitive. Exhalation, however, is not. Letting go of the breath involves intentionally contracting the abdominal muscles including the pelvic floor and releasing the breath upward.

The most common of the breath techniques is the Ujjayi (*ooh-jah-ee*). Ujjayi means victorious in Sanskrit, and it's typical to hear it called the ocean breath. Have you ever been in a yoga class and heard someone hissing through their nose like a cobra on steroids? Yeah, that's the Ujjayi. No, it doesn't have to be that fucking loud, but they think it makes them a "true" yogi. The ocean breath is a valving trick with the back of your throat. There's absolutely zero way for me to describe it in any manner here for you to use, but I'll give it a fucking shot. Think of your throat as the neck of a balloon. If you stretch the neck out, you can control the flow of air out of the balloon. Same goes for the ocean breath, except you're squeezing the back of your throat.

Yes, you can hear it when people are practicing. No, it shouldn't sound like a pit of vipers. While Prana is traditionally defined as life force, in physical yoga practice, it means breath. Ayama means to regulate or expand (in the Bhagavad Gita it literally means to halt. In this case, practioners mean hold. Retention.). Together, Pranayama is breathing in and out in a controlled way, the intake and release of the most vital fucking energy. There are a lot of different ways to breathe with a lot of different results.

For shits and giggles, here are some of them:

Bhramari (*brah-mar-ee*) - the humming bee breath.

Kapalabhati (*ka-pal-ab-hati*) - the skull shining breath[1]

Nadi Shodana (*nah-dee-show-dah-nuh*) - the purification breath involves breathing first through one nostril and then out through the other. (Not particularly my favorite but great if you have a migraine).

Agni-Prasana (*ah-g-nee-pr-ah-sah-na*) - the fire breath (this one is more common to Kundalini (*koon-dah-lee-nee*) yoga).

Bhastrika (*bha-stri-kaah*) - the bellows breath (designed to build energy and heat quickly).

Yeah, the breath is THAT important. Does it mean you can't practice yoga without mastering the breath? Hell no. I try to guide the breath and every so often in my general classes, we'll work together on the breath. But I typically limit close instruction on the Pranayama to my therapeutic yoga classes. I cue

1   Something about skull shining speaks to me.

breathing through your nostrils if you can, but recommend breathing in any case (it's surprising how often I have to remind clients to breathe).

Here's the deal. Our lungs are capable of a lot more capacity than most of us use. Each half of a pair of lungs is roughly the size of an American football. Physically, our lungs extend from our collarbones to below our ribs. A healthy person participating in vigorous exercise uses maybe seventy percent of their lung capacity. Running, cycling, and most other high-level cardio activities, create a shallow inhale into our upper chest allowing for a faster rhythm. Yoga breathing, when you're really focusing on it, can utilize almost one hundred percent of your lung capacity.

And remember, we breathe while we move. So not only are you increasing the length and balance of your breath, you're strengthening the muscles involved with breathing. Sometimes you're working against your diaphragm, other times, the intercostal muscles between the ribs. Stronger muscles mean better fucking performance. See where I'm going here? For me, yoga makes breathing more accessible. I'm not only focusing on breathing, I'm also widening my attention to both movement and breath. The rhythm becomes more fluid and, indeed intuitive, as muscle memory builds. This is the one area I will encourage muscle memory.

Breathing can be a sticking point. Yoga is a multilevel processing activity. You're thinking about where your feet are. You're thinking about which is left and right. You're thinking the person behind you can see exactly how large your ass is. Oh, that might only be me. My point is, spending more energy thinking about something that you do intuitively can feel like a goddamned nightmare.

This whole breathing thing is the fucking bomb. Total anecdotal evidence here for you quantitative minds out there: A few years ago, a doc diagnosed me with exercise-induced asthma. Personally, I thought it was an allergic reaction to all of the cardio. *Shrug*. Mind you, this news came well into my forties. I've run since I was a teenager. I just thought everyone had that "I might have a heart attack any minute" sheen when they exercised. My numbers during the lung capacity test showed up much higher than most asthma patients. The allergist willingly gave credit to my years of yoga breathing for the results. Cue the friggin' jokes about a lot of hot air—now.

Post-operative clients in my therapeutic classes have improved their oxygen numbers. One of my clients, originally from Poland, has COPD (Chronic Obstructive Pulmonary Disease) from a childhood bout of tuberculosis. She has increased her oxygen numbers and improved her lung capacity through yoga breathing. Even if you never step into a yoga class, it doesn't hurt to sit and take six or seven breaths as deeply as you can once a night. Oh, and don't smoke. I hear it's not good for you.

I'm going to drop some Harvard science on you. Deep breathing practice reduces stress. You know, it's that little thing we all deal with from time to time. Okay, I may experience a little road rage on occasion. Just barely. There are all kinds of technical terms for breathing practice; diaphragmatic breathing, abdominal breathing, and the classic paced breathing. It all boils down to one thing: shallow chest breathing increases anxiety, amplifies tension, and general pissiness. Deep rhythmic breathing slows your heart rate, lowers your blood pressure, and helps you relax. That's fucking Harvard Medical, people.[2]

Scientific evidence aside, it's not a huge leap to connect improved stress management skills, with a whole slew of improved ailments.[3] Learning to control our breath and practicing deep breathing reduces impulsivity. Remember when your parents said if you were mad, count to ten? Add ten full slow breaths and you literally can't stay angry. Not this metaphorical *literally* bullshit, but really. You won't be able to stay mad. Strong breathers improve their overall happiness and optimism. I don't know about you, but I can hit apocalyptic fury in one-point-two seconds. Taking a few deeps breaths brings me down a fucking notch or two.

---

2   Publications, Harvard Health. "Take a deep breath." *Harvard Health*, 2009, www.health.harvard.edu/staying-healthy/take-a-deep-breath. Accessed 9 Mar. 2017.
3   Publications, Harvard Health. "Relaxation techniques: Breath control helps quell errant stress response." *Harvard Health*, 18 Mar. 2016, www.health.harvard.edu/mind-and-mood/relaxation-techniques-breath-control-helps-quell-errant-stress-response. Accessed 22 Apr. 2017.

Daily breathing practice can reduce cravings and addictions. Now, don't go hog wild for the oxygen diet. I've tried the ten-breath thing to avoid that handful of almond M & Ms. In ten breaths, I still want the fucking M & Ms. But hey, it may work for you. It can't hurt. A deep breathing practice can help manage and reduce pain. Remember my shattered ankle? I have a little problem with opiate painkillers. I can't take them. They make me vomit. FOR FUCKING DAYS. Yeah, it's a bummer. I will say, some serious deep breathing can mitigate a lot. And perhaps a little medicinal herb helped too. Allegedly.

Deep breathing takes practice and can cause dizziness (you know, all of that oxygen pumping through your system). There is another side effect I've seen. Just as breathing can calm turbulent emotions, working closely with the breath can also trigger uncontrollable emotional responses. No fucking lie. This is akin to having your therapist tap your repressed memories like a keg. Get the Solo cups ready. Breathing can release pent up frustration, deep-seated sorrow, and unknown suppressed fear. I've had my fair share of clients burst into tears or have a momentary freak out during breathing practice.

Hence, the "I am breathing, bitch!" Hey, it's all good. Take a fucking breath.

CHAPTER 8

Did That Bitch Just Fart?

Type "yoga detox" into any search engine and you'll be rewarded with over eleven million hits. Eleven fucking MILLION. Poses to detox. Seasonal detox plans. Yoga diet detoxes. New Year's Yoga detoxes. Special sequences to detox. You know how many of those are science-based? ONE. One in the first five pages of hits. One lonely little science journal article. What is the world coming to? I'm going to go out on a realistic fucking limb here. Hey, I can mic drop like Stephen Hawking. Yoga CANNOT fucking DETOX your body.

You can't squeeze your liver. Nor can you rinse out your spinal fluid. Are you fucking kidding? You can't refresh your kidneys. Doing yoga cannot release toxins from your body. However, ANY physical exercise inducing sweat the day after over-imbibing will indeed encourage your body to process some fluids, BUT you must drink a lot of water to actually flush the system. And you can drink water without doing any workout at all, which is what typically happens. *Ah que la chingada! Ajúa!*[1]

Here's where I will go up against any yogi in defense of scientific research. Your liver is the natural fucking bouncer of your dance club. It works fine on its own. Your kidneys don't need to be massaged or flexed. It hurts my brain to even say it. The removal of toxins from your body happens naturally and automatically. Physical exercise improves one's overall health and thereby creates a more efficient process. Okay, your internal organs do need healthy nutrition and hydration in the form of water to really flex their muscles, but you don't need to massage them, twist them, wring them, or any other claim a yoga teacher might offer. Have I mentioned how friggin' amazing the human body is?

Treat your body right and it will treat you right. Most of the time.

In general, a balanced diet low in processed sugar, heavy on the fresh vegetables, and plenty of hydration is a good rule of thumb to stay healthy. Blah, blah, blah, I'm not saying anything you don't already know. Do I love me some juicing? Hell yes. Because I feel light and nourished; I'm talking super svelte and sexy. People always seem to remark how my skin glows when I'm sucking down my nutrient-packed seventy percent greens to thirty percent fruit concoctions. Maybe because I'm colossally packing the veggies and not nibbling on fried chicken. Maybe my skin glows because I sleep better. I sleep better because I'm not full of heavy food in need of energetic

---

1   Loosely translated this means Fucking A! Wahoo!

digestion. As a fucking detox? Nah.

Yoga can't do that either. Period. If yoga doesn't detoxify, what the fuck does it do to your insides?

It induces farting. Yes, I'm going to say it. We all pass gas. Women too. It should be noted that at least one person per yoga class farts. You can't stop it. We're bending, twisting, folding, and generally squeezing our bodies. It will promote the movement of air. Doesn't matter if you didn't eat beans last night. If you have any air hiding in your belly (and by belly, I mean intestines), you will fucking fart in yoga class.

Anecdotally, if you're having a weird digestion day, a strong twisting practice can set you up right as rain the next day. You're moving things around. Note, it is NOT a detox. It's just blood flow combined with a lot of moving and jiggling. And deep breathing. Did you read the "I AM Breathing, Bitch" chapter?

The tricky part of this farting business is some serious yogis will just let them rip. If a yoga teacher doesn't warn new folks, this can throw off the entire idea of a yoga class. My dental hygienist, also a yoga client of mine, quit going to a class because this one yogi fuckwit farted without regard the entire hour. And no matter where she moved her mat, he seemed to gravitate toward her. No one warned her. No one sniggered out loud. It was simply ignored because they were all "REAL" fucking yogis. Oh come on! Acknowledge, inform, and say the word fart. We're all grownups. Well, most of us are. Hey, don't look at me! She couldn't handle the indiscriminate farting. To be fair, she has three daughters, so her toot immunity is low.

I don't blame her. I know a lot of women who are mortified by the idea that they, just like everyone, fart. At home, I'm an unabashed tooter. Too much information, I know, but I have three offspring, two of whom are pseudo-adult men at the time of writing. If you have boys, you know they fart, cut the cheese, cut 'em, and burn 'em. When the kids were small there was nothing better, especially for the boys, than a great fart joke. I could embarrass my dotter[2] here. Let's just say you don't want to be closed up in a car with her unless it's equipped with automatic speed down windows. (Love you, Dotter!)

Of course, my darling hubby is a delicate fucking flower. He's very offended by the farting in our house. We mothers will tell you; once you have a baby all dignity gets thrown out the window. The veil has been parted. Hey, fellas, women fart. Get over it.

In public, of course, I adhere to polite norms and remove myself from mixed company. Not because I'm embarrassed to fart because it's common courtesy. Okay, it's a little embarrassing. Let's face it, one of the weird societal norms we have is our aversion to any natural bodily function. Burping,

2   This is an affectionate title bestowed upon my first-born offspring. I use it when I'm writing so as to keep her anonymous.

farting, menstruation, the list goes on and on. On the flip side, we love to make these bodily functions the butt of jokes. Farting in public is fucking taboo. Unlike when one of my sons walks into my office, drops one and books out in glee shouting, "It was Fintan!" Ha. Friggin' ha.

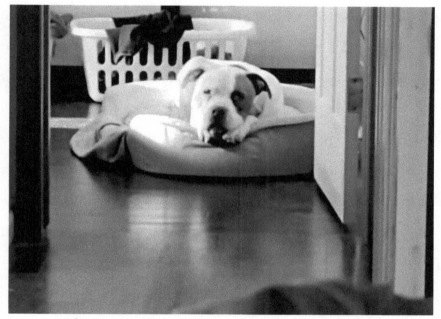

This is Fintan. He has one expression. Happy, sad, or guilty.

A yoga class is tough enough for some people to join, but add farting to the mix and they may never try again. I warn people passing gas is a possible side effect of practicing. Everyone laughs and blushes, but someone is going to fart. If I need to pass gas, I do without fucking fanfare or drama. It is, after all, entirely natural and almost impossible to control, especially when you're on your back hugging your knees to your chest. A little word of advice? The more you resist, the louder it will be.

So yoga doesn't detox but does cause farting. Why the hell am I asking you to give it a shot? That might not feel like enough on which to hang a practice. A regular yoga practice can actually change your physical wellbeing and that statement IS supported by fucking science.[3] Pages and pages of scientifically proven benefits of a healthy, mindful yoga practice exist. There's nothing esoteric about it. Many vinyasa flow classes and Ashtanga practices can crank your heart rate up in the aerobic range. Even if you're not boosting into the "Wow, I'm really working here" range, regular yoga practice can improve your cardiovascular health and lower your resting heart rate. As outlined in the chapter "I Am Breathing, Bitch" yoga can increase your overall oxygen intake, which improves your aerobic conditioning. It's an exponential and fabulous loop.

The most obvious benefit is improved strength and flexibility.

Regular yoga practice can increase your circulation. Inverted poses encourage stronger blood flow because you're fighting gravity. No, you are not increasing the blood flow to your upper extremities. Your cardiovascular system is closed. If it is open, you're bleeding out and get thy fucking self to a hospital. I'm going to hop on my soapbox here.

---

3   "Yoga: What You Need To Know." Edited by INna Belfer and David Shirtleff, *National Center for Complementary and Integrative Health*, U.S. Department of Health and Human Services, 2018, www.nccih.nih.gov/health/yoga-what-you-need-to-know.

You do not increase the amount of blood in the brain by being upside down. I like a good prasarita padottanasa (*prah-sar-e-tah pah-doe-tah-nah-sah*) (wide-angle standing forward fold) as much as the next person but I've also seen a lot of murder shows, and torture almost always includes hanging upside down by your ankles. TORTURE. For all kinds of reasons, the brain likes stability. Too much or too little blood flow can cause damage to the arteries, broken blood vessels, and dun dun duhhhhh . . . death by stroke.

Okay, back to oxygen. The thing about better circulation is you're improving your oxygen delivery system. Think about oxygen for a sec.

Better oxygen intake via a more efficient breath, coupled with improved blood flow, allows all of the systems requiring oxygen, to be fueled at a higher rate. Low oxygen levels affect brain function. Guess what? That's a bad thing. Low blood oxygen can disturb your quality of sleep, weaken your immune system, and impact your blood pressure. I don't know about you, but if I'm sleeping poorly, somebody is in fucking mortal peril. The mental benefits lead to physical benefits.

I teach a Tuesday evening class at 7:30 p.m. Yes, it's pretty close to my bedtime. When people ask me to describe that class I say, "It's Last One to Bed Is A Rotten Egg yoga." I'm dipping into "Zen and The Art of Chocolate Cake" here, but a little bite won't hurt. Evening Yoga in my world is ooey gooey, fantastic stretchy yoga. The lights are low. The music is groovy (yes, I still use that word) and the flow is all about taking the energy down.

Combine all of that with the deep, rhythmic breath and woosh! Final relaxation is a fast pass to groggyville. Hence, *last one to bed is a rotten egg*. No fucking lie. Folks who can't sleep to save their souls, let alone their family, sack out on a yoga mat on a wood floor in a studio with a bunch of strangers. We're talking snoring, drooling slumber. Don't worry, I never leave them there.

Point is, effective cardiovascular health combined with higher oxygen levels and a more powerful breath, lead to the ability to shut down the noise in your brain and doze.

Wait, I'm not fucking done. All of the same rules apply to an energetic practice, except the snoozing. Sure, you may fart once in a while in class, but after all of that synchronous moving, breathing, and non-thinking, you're going to be floating out of class in a mood even the rudest dickweed at the grocery store can't ruin. They can park you in so closely you'll have to climb through the fucking back hatch to get to the driver's seat and you'll still be hunky-dory. Maybe you'll post a picture on Facebook or Instagram tagging them as douchebag assholes BUT you won't key their cars.

Seriously, I didn't key their cars. Fucking yoga! Thank you very much.

Well, hell for breakfast! I've just proved that yoga CAN detox something. Yoga can detoxify a shitty, fucking attitude. Mindful awareness, deep breathing, ignoring the farters, and improving your overall health can improve your mood. To give credit, almost all exercises releases endorphins or endogenous cannabinoids depending on the current research you're citing. These chemicals, if you didn't know, are the exact same ones released when you eat chocolate, orgasm, chow on spicy foods, smoke a doobie, or pet puppies. Endorphins and endogenous cannabinoids are neurotransmitters that help regulate the central and autonomic nervous systems, the immune system, endocrine network, and reproductive system.

Seriously, your body creates its own fucking opiates AND cannabinoids! Have I mentioned how friggin' amazing the human body is? No one person has the same endocrine response. You know what, bitches? Meditation releases endorphins and endogenous cannabinoids, too.

Think about it. Yoga is active meditation. Wait for it . . . here's the kicker; yoga scientifically demonstrates a higher efficacy in improving mental wellness and emotional stability than ANY other fucking exercise.

The combination of physical movement, mental focus, and deep breathing reduces anxiety and diminishes the symptoms of chronic depression at the same levels that cognitive behavioral therapy does. I'm not knocking therapy. Believe me, some of the peeps in this house have only survived because of some seriously fabulous therapists. When one of the offspring asks me why I see a therapist I say, "Because it reduces my urge to murder you in your sleep." They always agree that's a good idea. Heck, Son 1 has toyed with the idea of becoming a psychologist. No jokes about crazy fucking mothers, please. BUT, yoga does affect and improve balance in brain chemistry. BAM! Oh, and that HAS been proven scientifically. I don't make this shit up.

Besides, if yoga can chill out this Aztec Mexican Apache, imagine what it can do for you with a little practice.

CHAPTER 9

My Dog Doesn't Do Downward

Almost every conversation I have about my professional life goes like this:

"What do you do?"

"I'm a writer."

"Oh, I've always wanted to write a book."

OR

"What do you do?"

"I teach yoga."

"I know yoga is supposed to be good for you, but I'm not very flexible."

Even after thirty-plus years of yoga, I still find room for more flexibility and strength. You will never increase flexibility unless you change what you're doing. I know I'm repeating myself, but sometimes you have to hear information more than once to absorb it. Yoga is an opportunity to become better acquainted with your body. Not the body you had twenty years ago.

Not the body you would like to have. The body you have, right this minute. And it took a lifetime to arrive at this particular moment.

We've gained weight. We've lost weight. We might have had a baby or babies. Maybe we have been ill or injured. If you're a regular runner, biker, or hiker you have different issues than swimmers or tennis players or hockey players. It will take time to become familiar with the body you have right now. It will take patience and persistence to make changes significant enough to notice.

Yoga is the long con.

I have a regular client who's been coming to my class for about ten years now. He's a runner. Not like I'm a plodder, but a real runner. He races and runs half marathons and shit. He actually convinced me to run in a 5K a few years back . . . oh man. It was the first race I'd run since the eighth grade. Tragic story. It was the last time I ever ran in an official capacity. Boo-hoo. I didn't stop running. I simply prefer to run with my dogs. The point is, my client the runner, had been doggedly coming to yoga class. When he started, he couldn't touch his shins in a forward fold never mind touching his toes. A lot of athletes—I'm talking active, healthy athletes—can't touch their toes to save their lives. Large, powerful muscles tend to be short. That's why they're large and powerful. Big muscles are also hefty.

Have I mentioned yet how yoga is about learning to control your own body weight? Oh, okay, yoga is also about learning to control your own body weight. This is also a tenet of Pilates, another passion of mine, but we're talking yoga. Think about your head. Terrible sentence. Think about the skull and the brain. Including all of the soft bits, your head weighs approximately eleven pounds. Are you thinking about it? Find a ten-pound bowling ball and hold it in one hand. Just hold it. Heavy, heh?

Your skin is actually the heaviest part of your body weighing in at about 24 pounds. I'm talking just your fucking skin. Not even counting the extra ten or twenty pounds you might be carrying. Okay, me, I'm carrying the extra weight.

Flexibility refers to the range of motion in a joint and the length of the muscles across those joints that control movement.

Fact: flexibility is a result of multiple factors, not the least of which, is bone structure. Some people have better range of motion in a joint than others because their bones are shaped differently. You can control or maneuver some of the other factors, but the shape of your skeletal structure ain't one.

Fact: Age is an element of range of motion. The older you grow, the less naturally flexible you become. Let's face it: shit starts drying out.

Fact: Biological sex plays a role in flexibility. In general, females have leaner muscle fibers than men, hence their muscles don't get as short. Bulky, strong muscles are shorter than leaner, strong muscles. Sorry, fellas. That doesn't mean female muscles don't get tight. They do. Males tend to be less flexible. The greater the muscle density (how big your guns are), the more limited your range of motion. Flexible muscles aren't necessarily weak, but they are longer and leaner. Remember Big Jim and his friends? (Chapter 3: Yoga Ain't for Sissies)?

Remember, yoga is the long con. In my experience, it takes about three months to get comfortable on the mat. (Learning the lingo of a particular teacher; figuring out which limb goes where; getting into the habit of going to yoga class in the first place.) Add another three months to really get in the groove. (Learning what pose is which; remembering left from right even when you're upside down; and running out of fucks to give if anyone else is looking at you.) It's right about the sixth or seventh month mark you realize you've gained some range of movement. It sneaks up on you.

It's about that benchmark when you begin to feel stronger in certain poses. You might move from a modified plank to full plank. Or maybe something I've said or shown you fifty times suddenly clicks, and you move forward in your practice. Thirty-plus years I've practiced yoga, and I can't do the sidesplits. I couldn't do them when I was seven years old. I don't have the room between my greater Trochanter, or maybe my lesser Trochanter—I don't really know or care—and my acetabulum. In plain speak, I strike bone on bone before I'm ever close to the splits.

I have zero interest in doing the splits. It's not something I'm dying to add to my resume. I can do, after thirty years of practice, Urdhva Dhanurasana (*oord-vah don-your-ahs-anna*) (wheel pose). It's a fancy name for a back bend. And I will tell you, sixty percent of accomplishing the asana, was mental. Fear. Fear held me out of that pose for thirty years. One day I thought, "Fuck it." That was the day I found it. It's an ego pose. I feel like a sassy yoga bitch whenever I do it.

The thing about flexibility is it's flexible. Heh heh hehe. Seriously, I don't care what mojo jojo someone touts about gaining flexibility fast; remember it's a patience game. All of my yoga practices include warming up. Getting the body moving a little before you ask it to give you something. A healthy yoga flow, as I studied in Viniyoga, eases you into an energetic pose and then backs you out of it.

In an hour-long yoga practice, I include three to five minutes of light meditative suggestions, clearing the cobwebs and connecting to breath. After that, ten minutes of warming up with movement designed to support the stronger poses coming later in the flow. As I add poses to build the flow, I cue the lower energy version of poses first. The flow repeats with the opportunity to move into the stronger forms. The bulk of vigorous movement lasts thirty to thirty-five minutes, and then we cool down which includes some deeper stretching and finding our way into savasana. While most classes are typically an hour, a seventy-five-minute class would be my ideal.

And be honest, how many of you take even ten minutes of stretching after a hard workout? Don't lie. I know you don't. I'm a fitness teacher. I see you. You're the person who thinks the last fifteen minutes of my Fit Fun Flex class is really for booking out early to hit the grocery store on the way home. Maybe you're the person in my cycle class who ignores the ten minutes of stretch I guide to squeeze in that extra twenty-calorie burn or two miles or whatever. You are definitely the person who thinks, "Ah, this bitch is cracked if she thinks I'm going to waste ten or fifteen minutes of my precious time stretching."

Sure as shit, that's often the person complaining of lower back pain or shoulder issues or sciatic pain because stretching is for sissies. You're damn right, this bitch stretches. On average, I do six to seven hours of yoga a week and I'm STILL tight as fuck some days. I teach twelve hours of fitness. And I think I've pointed out I'm not willowy or lissome. I'm a friggin' Rhino! Fact: unless you've been doing yoga since you were four years old every day for hours, you're never as flexible as you'd like to be. (Think of training like a Cirque Du Soleil star or a contortionist.)

Even if you're not a world-famous Gumby impersonator, flexibility is the Swiss army knife of health. Let me count the ways.

The longer the fibers in your muscles, the more strength you can gain in those muscles. Strong muscles can reduce the loss of bone density, particularly important as we earn more years. Grow wiser. Age like fine wine. You get the idea. Along that line, in addition to strong, lean muscles reducing the risk of injury during any activity, flexible muscles and a good range of motion prevent age-related breaks. And we're not getting any younger. Lean, flexible muscles mean easier blood circulation. Better circulation improves your immune system and healing time. Um, better circulation can reduce the risk of all sorts of degenerative diseases. Better circulation means better oxygen delivery. Lean, flexible muscles also mean more flexible arterial walls, which reduce the risk of heart attack and stroke.

Speaking as a woman who will never be slender, longer, leaner muscles help maintain weight. Gaining longer, leaner muscles can translate into fewer inches. While I've not lost a pound practicing yoga, I have maintained my weight.

Strong, lean muscles help you maintain better posture. No, you don't fucking shrink with age. Okay, you do SORT OF shrink with age. As you get older, things dry out. The fluid in the discs in our vertebrae does become a smidgen denser, thus, reducing—just barely—the length of your spine. Your arches might flatten as you grow older, and some of us are at greater risk for osteoporosis. Hey, gravity is a bitch. But mostly, you lose muscle strength in your core (those are your abs) and you end up slouching. Bad posture.

Guess what? Exercise, and yes, I mean YOGA, can prevent and improve all of those conditions. Well, it can't prevent some things from drying out, but it can improve your core strength, which in turn can keep your spine longer and healthier. Building stronger, leaner muscles prevents bone loss and can increase bone density, which helps to prevent or delay osteoporosis.

Do you need more? No? Good, cuz that's all I've got at the moment.

CHAPTER 10

Yoga Pants? Oh Hell No.

I broached the concept of this book with friends at one of our regular salons. Many of the chapter titles ended up in drunken dry erase marker on my fridge. It's a process and we have a good time. The topics of being overweight and out of shape rolled around. We're not dainty people. Seriously. We enjoy our food and booze.

I hear it more than I would like. Can you do yoga if you're overweight? Well, this is a bullshit question for me. Define overweight. At the time of writing, I'm hanging onto twenty extra pounds above my ideal weight. I'm also of a particular age when my metabolism isn't on my top ten list. I'm a fan of the Paleo-style diet. My cousin David sends me all kinds of caveman jokes. Diverticulitis and Celiac run in my father's family. My daughter has a full-blown wheat allergy as well as our Native American-genetic intolerance to dairy. Paleo treats me right. Does that mean I'm currently in Paleo mode? No.

The particular age I'm at is also the "Out of Fucks to Give" age. Paleo takes work I'm not into devoting at this juncture of my life's road. Getting into a size ten that's probably really a size eight, isn't floating my boat any longer. Oh, I have my days, but my hubby hasn't kicked me out of bed yet. He likes to say, "You're a hearty woman, honey." He's still alive. Even at my thinnest, I'm not a tiny woman. And you know what? I don't have any desire to be. I look like I could break someone in two. Ahimsa. Ahimsa. (Ahimsa is the act of non-harm.) I'm working on it.

I teach ten hours of fitness a week, and five to six hours of yoga. Out of those five hours of yoga, one hour is a serious energy burn. The rest is a combination of cycle classes, and a class that contains a little bit of everything; Zumba, cardio, weights, and core work. This is me reminding myself that I'm fit.

For those of you who like to count, according to a Harvard Medical School study1 on exercise, a person in a typical yoga class will burn approximately ten percent of their body weight in calories per half an hour. Fine, I'll math for you. If you weigh one-hundred-sixty pounds, you'll burn one-hundred-sixty calories in thirty minutes of Hatha yoga. Hatha yoga being the lowest key, stretching type. Now, I'm rounding numbers for the sake of easy math and let's say that's my Beginning yoga class.

1 Publications, Harvard Health. "Calories burned in 30 minutes for people of three different weights." *Harvard Health*, www.health.harvard.edu/newsweek/Calories-burned-in-30-minutes-of-leisure-and-routine-activities.htm. Accessed 17 Feb. 2017.

My classes break down roughly the same: five to seven minutes of Pratyahara (prah-tee-ah-har-ah) and Dharana, followed by five to seven minutes of warm-up (we'll count those), thirty to forty minutes of vinyasa (including cool down), and finishing with seven to ten minutes of savasana. For every class, you're getting roughly forty minutes of calorie burning. This is one reason why in my ideal world, yoga classes would be seventy-five minutes. The energy of the practice in my Vinyasa Flow class is amped well up into the cardio range and the energy of my Evening Yoga is cranked way down.

Based on someone weighing 160 pounds, I would estimate any vigorous yoga; say a vinyasa flow or an Ashtanga-style practice, raises the calorie burn into the two-twenty range. That's four hundred calories burned in forty minutes of yoga practice. Nothing to sneeze at, right? That covers the workout aspect of yoga, but I'm repeating a caveat. In all of the years I've practiced, I cannot qualitatively attribute any of my weight loss to yoga.

Understanding my body through the relationship of yoga helps me stay in touch with all other aspects of my physical condition. Research shows yoga helps you maintain your weight, which I have experienced.[2] I may have gained the twenty pounds in those two years of dealing with injury, but since

2 Bouchez, Colette. "Yoga for Weight Loss?" Edited by Louise Chang, *WebMD*, WebMD, July 2006, www.webmd.com/fitness-exercise/features/yoga-for-weight-loss#1. Accessed 17 Feb. 2017.

then I haven't gained a single pound. Fuck if I've lost a single pound either, shrug.

Pretty safe to say, we all feel ten pounds over our ideal weight, and we perceive that we look heavier than we are. We are sold those ideas from a multibillion-dollar industry invested in keeping us unhappy with who we are and how we look. Sure, I'm not at my ideal body weight, but my blood pressure is lower than average, my bloodwork always comes back ridiculously healthy, and I can teach ten fitness classes a week and get out of bed every morning without too much muss or fuss. A double espresso helps.

I see a significant difference in some of my poses between now and my thinner weight. Not in my flexibility, but in my comfort level in the pose. Try a friggin' halasana (plow pose: feet over head) with a generous D-cup bosom. Twenty pounds ago, halasna was easier. That does not mean poses are inaccessible to me. Remember, yoga—particularly my flavor of yoga—is about controlling body weight. If you're a strong, fit person who weighs more than the undernourished, skin and bone models we're being sold as the ideal body type, then you can do yoga. Yoga is about balance and core strength as much as it is about flexibility. Even the skinnies have issues with yoga if they don't have any muscle strength.

Remember, flexibility has as much to do with body mechanics and range of motion as stretching does.

Also, yoga is a mind game. Remember my story about wheel pose (it's called urdhva dhanurasana)? Right now I'm in the market to tackle a headstand (salamba sirsasana – *sah-lom-bah shear-shahs-anna*). I have the strength and core power to accomplish it if I could only get my attachment out of the way. I'm attached to the fear of falling. Go figure. Svadhyaya (*svahd-yah-yah*) is one of the Niyamas. Part of svadhyaya is accepting and welcoming our limitations, so I'm working on it.

If you're not fit, no matter what size, physical activity will be a challenge. If you haven't stretched a minute of your life yoga will be a challenge. The physical benefits of a healthy, mindful yoga practice alone are worth the discomfort you'll feel in a yoga class. And I'll call out the bullshit yoga in most studios that's marked as a thin, white woman sport. I avoid looking at the various yoga magazines that showcase only perfect yoga bodies on their covers. I have family in the photography business. A long time ago, my uncle showed me how advertisement photos featuring young, skinny women are manipulated for the right look.

Profiles are airbrushed. Ribs are shortened or lengthened. For fucks sake, belly buttons get repositioned for perfect placement and by perfect, I mean perfectly rubbish. Thighs are made thinner, smoother. Thigh gap? NOT NORMAL, unless you're teeny tiny or undernourished or have a great digital touch-up artist.

In *Beautiful Girls*, screenwriter, Scott Rosenberg gave Rosie O'Donnell the most brilliant monologue of modern film, as far as I'm concerned. It begins with fabulous details about the dangers of a certain music television channel, porn magazines, and advertising agencies. "Girls with big tits have big asses. Girls with little tits have little asses. God doesn't fuck around. He's a fair guy. He gave the fatties big, beautiful tits and the skinnies little tiny nigglers.[3] It's not my rule. If you don't like it, call Him." You don't have to take my word for it. YouTube it.

We don't need any help thinking we're inadequate. The bottom line is fear. And shit heads. Assholes can ruin everything. And let me tell you, there are Buddhist, Zen, yoga assholes out there aplenty. Find a place where real people, real practitioners of not only sound yoga practice, but of kindness, will welcome you and help you on your path.

Listen, they come into my class. If you've ever been in a gym you know whom I'm speaking about. Man or woman in the chic work out clothes, hair done or the perfect messy bun, the cutesy yoga mat, and probably every fucking alignment issue that makes me cringe. And thin; I guarantee it. They trot into the studio sure of one of two things; they'll be the class favorite because their yoga is perfect, or they know infinitely more than I do. Or both.

---

3   For those of you who just raised an outraged eyebrow, calm down. Niggle means trifle, as in a trifling sum i.e., small, tiny, or teeny.

I tamp down my Apache ancestry and go to my Zen accepting place. I peel off my top layer and their faces fall. I am not the slender, picture perfect yoga instructor from the cover of a magazine. I'm a muscled, curvy, tattooed harlot. However, my yoga kung fu is strong. Their response to my practice can go a couple of ways. They either bristle at my corrections on their perfect yoga form and never come back. Or they drop their hoity-toity attitude, and join our yoga tribe. These true yogis roll their eyes when I talk about length AND strength and then, they make an adjustment I've been nagging about. I see the minute it happens because suddenly yoga is challenging and difficult for them.

Yes, this is me judging. I've taken the gamut of classes in every type of location imaginable; beach yoga, recreation center yoga, and yoga studios of all ilk. These misinformed yoga yahoos are everywhere and scarily some of them are teachers. Bottom line, no matter the entire yoga philosophy; no matter Hindu, Buddhist, Christian, or Islam; no matter scrawny or zaftig; blue, black, brown, or white . . . oh man, I'd be blue (have you seen *The Fifth Element?* I digress) yoga is gracious and welcoming. If you don't feel gladly received, then fuck 'em. They're probably full of shit and not worth your time.

So when *those* types come into my class, I smile warmly. I offer my brand of yoga with grace and kindness. Oh, I may grumble when I get home, but as the saying goes, "You can lead a horse to water . . ." The people who join the tribe have experienced a paradigm shift and have re-discovered yoga. Have I mentioned it's awesome?

You don't need fancy yoga clothes. Hell, half the time I teach class in my pajamas—very comfortable, non-holey pajamas. As long as I can move in them, I will wear them on the mat. Men, a tuckable t-shirt, if you care (I don't) and some light sweatpants or shorts will work. Please don't go commando. Did I mention tasers yet? I will later. Ladies, a comfortable sports bra or tank top with a shelf bra, comfortable pants or shorts, and yes, the commando rule applies to you, too. Sure, yoga pants are fine (and many don't need underwear), but they are unnecessary. I do like capris, whether they're running tights or yoga pants or sweatpants. Frankly, I'm short. Okay, I'm average, but remember my rant about thin white women? Yoga pants tend to be long on me. They get in the way. Layer up because it might get hot and savasana is definitely a cool down.

Oh, and always shop the clearance rack.

If togging out in a cute yoga outfit does it for you, motivates you, and gets you in the damn studio, then by all means tog. But it's not a prerequisite to get in the door.

CHAPTER 11

Namaste Bitches

You've heard it and you may even have said it at the closing of a yoga class. In the scope of this discussion, it can sum up the entire cultural appropriation of not only a living, dynamic philosophy, but also of a prolific, contemporary religion with approximately 1.2 BILLION adherents. Okay, I'm gonna bend some folks out of shape right now. Heh heh, get it? It might be a bumpy ride. Buckle up. It's how I roll.

Even though it's not a religion, yoga has an integral relationship with both Hinduism (yes, a religion) and Buddhism (no, not a religion; a practice). Just for giggles, Hinduism (with the aforementioned 1.2 billion participants) is one of the three most prolific religions in the world. Christianity has two billion adherents while Islam has 1.6 billion. So we're not talking peanuts here.

There's no getting around the topic of the colonization and the subjugation of India from the mid-1700s that led to the eventual partitioning of India and Pakistan in 1947. That's two hundred years of European war, occupation, disregard, mistreatment, and marginalization, not to mention outlawing many Hindu and yoga practices. It's a lot of baggage.

I have the fortune of knowing some South Asian Indians. From India. They friggin' hate Namaste. Interestingly, they hate it for different reasons.

Namaste, or Namaskar in Sanskrit, literally means salutations or prostration. At the most basic level, it's Aloha. It's hello. It's Ní hǎo. It's Hola. It's a traditional greeting. In many Indian cultures, depending on region and caste (and there are many . . . seriously, it's a vast and varied country), greeting people includes bowing to elders and touching the elders' feet. I've seen this performed as a two-handed prostration (Dandavat). I've seen it practiced as a bow with a touch of the feet with one hand and a touch of the brow with the other (a form of Namaskar). This tradition is called the pranama (the last *a* is silent). It's a form of respect and honor.

Unlike yoga or Buddhism (there is plenty of discussion on this count), Hinduism IS a religion. Namaste is an element of the Hindu faith. The way it is treated in most western yoga classes is at best, a trite and empty gesture. At worst, in some of the more hippy dippy atmospheres, it is kind of a shot to the kneecaps of the religion. Looking at the deeper intrinsic meanings in both philosophical yoga and the tenets of Hinduism, namaha can be translated as *not mine; the release of ego in the presence of the One Truth, or the supreme spirit.*

So it can be a pretty big deal. It's similar to the way some people may use "Praise the Lord" in a church service, or "The Lord Be With You."

Another context where Namaste is used is in the practice of Bhakti yoga. Not typically a physical practice (though it can be), Bhakti yoga is considered a yoga of devotion. One of the more well-known teachers of this branch of yoga was Swami Sivananda. He considered Bhakti yoga "to soften the heart and remove jealousy, hatred, lust, anger, egoism, pride, and arrogance. It infuses joy, divine ecstasy, bliss, peace, and knowledge. All cares, worries and anxieties, fears, mental torments, and tribulations entirely vanish. The devotee is freed from the Samsaric wheel of birth and death. He attains the immortal abode of everlasting peace, bliss, and knowledge."1 In the case of a Bhakti meditation session, Namaste sometimes does close the practice.

You might hear it discussed in terms of universal oneness: *the divinity in me, sees and recognizes the divinity in you.* I'm gonna step out on my limb again—that's a lot of hoogety fucking boogety. Not bad hoogety boogety, but hooey nonetheless. That is the kind of pseudo hippy claptrap that irritates me. No, it's not very Zen to be irritated by things, but releasing attachment is a work in process. It's also common to hear from people who studied yoga in India that they have never heard Namaste uttered in any class or the context of any yoga practice. This smacks of the exoticization of a culture.

---

1   Burgin, Timothy. "Bhakti Yoga: the Yoga of Devotion • Yoga Basics." *Yoga Basics*, 1 Apr. 2020, www.yogabasics.com/learn/bhakti-yoga-the-yoga-of-devotion/.

It didn't start with us. As early as 1659, the French physician and philosopher François Bernier compared the "*jauguis* to the mystical practices of the occultists in Europe."[2] Basically, likening early yogis to astrologers, mediums, and fortunetellers. When we wrap up MTPY in the gossamer wings of butterflies and fluffer-doodles, we reinforce the worst kind of cultural appropriation. We continue the tradition of promoting yoga as "the embodiment of the sacred, mystical, and ecstatic dimensions of experience."[3] I get it. No matter your spiritual lean, I think we all fancy the idea of belonging to something bigger than ourselves.

I think the general, western yoga world is still caught up in the esoteric loop created by occultist Aleister Crowley, occultist Maud Allan, and the "White Light Yogi" Victor Dane, and Indra Devi. Since the mid-nineteenth century, there has been a push and pull between the practical and the traditional. Even before Krishnamacharya's influence on MTPY, the boundaries between true yoga and physical yoga had already been blurred. So you understand my irritation when I hear yoga people spout on about the holy yoga this and the sacred yoga that.

The problem at this point is where does appropriation stop and appreciation start.

---

2   Vernier, F. 1688. Memoire de Mr. Bernier sur le Qui'tisme des Indes. *Histoire des Ouvrages des Sçavanst* (September), art. V: 47-52
3   Singleton, Mark. *Yoga Body: the Origins of Modern Posture Practice.* Oxford University Press, 2010.

I have to refer back to my "What the Fuck IS Yoga" chapter. I've tried to give you the tiniest of idea; an amuse bouche, of what the banquet table of yogic philosophy includes. I like my limb so here I go again to say we can practice physical yoga separately from the core philosophy. After all, that it how *Hatha* yoga was originally considered by the Gheranda Samhita and Swami Vivekananda.[4] The ship has sailed in terms of calling it something other than yoga. Later, we'll talk modern transnational physical yoga, but for now yoga is yoga. I'm humbly mindful of the larger scope and I do work on things like ahimsa (non-harm), which is also a Buddhist and Hindu tenet . . . and Christian btw. Oh yeah? Revisit Luke 6:31. It's about doing unto others as you would have them do unto you; it's gotta a real *love your enemies* vibe. Pretty sure that means grace and kindness, people.

It's not an understatement to say modern yoga has been white-ified. Cultural appropriation is a complex and volatile topic whether it's yoga; Native American customs (a stern discussion about headdresses as concert attire was had here at home); dreadlocks (my awesome cousin rocks the dreads with his African/Mexican heritage but I'm a huera who shouldn't); food; or music, etc. It's true that yoga has been packaged and marketed as a product so much that the original tenets of Hatha have been stripped for

---

4   The GhS is a text that defines the earliest foundations of Yoga in Hinduism and Swami Vivekananda wrote one of the first English reimagnings (because it wasn't a literal translation) of Patanjali's *Yoga Sutras*.

the most part. One could say I'm guilty of packaging and marketing my own product in the form of this book. Meh.

I don't have an easy answer. I venerate the origins and philosophies while I'm teaching what is probably considered white woman yoga. Or in this case, Mexican/Apache/white woman yoga. I have a few tattoos all in the Asian style. I also have a Ganesha on my foot, which is a huge no-no. Maybe I'm on the wrong side of things; it's a wiggly line.

BUT I love yoga. I would love to see more people take up the practice as a physical activity that they can do for a lifetime. I try to offer bits and bobs of ahimsa, pratyahara (which is moving awareness from the external to the internal), dharana (in my class we focus on the union of breath and body), and dhyana (non-focus) during savasana. I don't regularly use the Sanskrit because I teach in middle-class, white America. They don't come to me for fancy. I like to think they enjoy my lack of bullshit, which I can truthfully say I practice in service of satya (Honesty).

As a yoga teacher, Pilates teacher, and fitness instructor, I am in service to my clients. In the spirit of ahimsa, if I adjust my classes to accommodate, to correct, and to inform, I work in service of their well-being and health. If they get my jokes, it's a bonus. I draw a pretty good crowd to my yoga classes. My fitness classes not so much. It's the balls to the wall mentality of western fitness. Faster, heavier, more. I'm not that teacher. If I amp things up so people feel the burn to get them to come back to my classes, I am not serving their greater good. Frankly, I've seen teachers who do more harm than help in the name of a great workout.

There's a fine balance between appropriation, parody, and homage. I don't honestly know where I come out at the end of most days. I would like to live in a world where expression of appreciation for a culture isn't a debate. At the same time, I totally respect the frustration.

I don't expect every client to embrace the whole of yoga. It's a little bonus when clients say, "Until your class, I've never been able to lie still in savasana." Or "I hate to meditate, but sometimes in your class I feel I'm right on the edge of having it click." I've even heard, "I was worried. You're a bit of a Chatty Cathy, but you got right down to business and you know your yoga." Introducing people to the eight-limbed path isn't my scene and there are many more qualified people out there from whom to learn.

I hope people will discover this amazing vessel we travel in and figure out how to treat themselves with ahimsa. Perhaps when we've all found that path, we can embrace it for everyone around us whether they have opposing political and religious beliefs, love differently than we do, or listen to Death Metal. (I love me some people who love Death Metal or maybe it's Black Metal; it's some kind of Metal. One of my darlings has even asked me to offer a Metal yoga class. No, nope, nah, sorry . . . uh-uh. Metal happens to ignite everything within me that is opposite of yoga. But I love them just the same.)

And the beautiful thing is, they love me back. Well, the say they do. They do. I'm pretty sure they do.

I like the definition of Namaste as a response to generosity. It's common in some regions as a guest's reply to hospitality. This one resonates with me. It's pretty damn generous of folks to make time in their day to come and hang with me. If you haven't realized yet, I'm not the most Zen of yoga instructors. Nor the most conventional. Whether it's a laid-back Saturday, or 6:15 on a Monday morning, people join me in the community of practice and show me kindness by not booing me out of the fucking room. Okay, some of them never come back and dive behind the aisles at the grocery store (again, small town) when they see me. So yes, I do offer a bow at the end of my class in fucking gratitude for their support.

But I don't Namaste.

CHAPTER 12

Yoga Teachers Need Tasers

Yoga class, with a covey of people, is a communal enterprise. Theoretically, you attend a class to benefit from the teacher's wisdom and instruction. The group setting can inspire and motivate you. I freely admit to adjusting a practice to address my physicality and philosophy when taking a class from another instructor. I may slow down a bit if the flow is moving too quickly by my measure. I will definitely ignore any alignment corrections or cues that directly contradict my grounding in Viniyoga. I invariably take seated meditation during final relaxation because I haven't attended a class outside of the Viniyoga practices besides my own that honor a full savasana.

I don't go into a studio and do my own thing. That's just rude.

It would be similar to attending a church service and during a hymn breaking out into Panic! At The Disco's "Hallelujah." Don't get me wrong, I dig independent thinking, but marching to your own beat in a class you've voluntarily joined kind of deflates the vibe. Remember, yoga isn't a religion, and you won't go to hell for practicing. It is, however, a merging of energy and common purpose. It's part of the Zen. I try not to talk much once we all get into the groove of a vinyasa. Remember the Orator Yoga Nazi? It spoils the mood.

Yes, a yoga class is a welcoming environment that should allow you to feel comfortable and relaxed. As relaxed as you can be. I've already ranted about Yoga Nazis in their various incarnations. I want you in my class. That said, there are polite niceties that most people observe for the benefit of the many. In every movie theater, on every plane (I was trying to talk quietly), or in every store, some folks just don't recognize their greater surroundings and the social graces that allow a society as large as ours to function smoothly. They are ignorant of their absolute talent at irksomeness.

Here's where my Zen slips for so many reasons.

I have a couple of regular clients who move at a slower pace than even I'm mapping. It's all good. They typically hover around the edge or corners of the studio, and it doesn't disrupt anyone's mojo. A colleague of mine attends my classes and sometimes moves faster or throws in an extra asana. They respect the flow and follow along without imposing on anyone around them. I take it as a gesture of respect that they come to my class, especially when they have their own classes to teach during the week. They aren't rattling the vibe.

I've experienced instances where a new face comes to class, and rather than adjusting to the vinyasa we're all channeling as a group, they decide to do their own thing in order to fit their practice. They run their own vinyasa at their own pace, typically flinging their bodies around pell-mell. Twice now, I've had these people plop their mats right in front of me. Talk about rage issues.

I soldiered on and tried to restore the groove, but Jesus and tacos, it was a shit show. No one in class could concentrate on not-concentrating. Several people fell, which happens less often than you think. I almost fell a couple of times. The general look on people's faces read, "Why aren't you jumping this bitch?" And the rogue clients in question remained absolutely unaware of the hostility radiating from the group. Someone later asked if we were being punk'd.

There's no winning in this kind of situation. Class must go on. Calling these people out in front of the group would be unprofessional and downright mean. We all focused on ignoring the wacky hodgepodge on display, but if I didn't address it, I could lose regular clients. I assured the folks who contacted me I would handle it the best way I knew how. Sure, it meant having to struggle through another class where we were all off kilter.

I politely waylaid these clients individually after class and gave the same exact speech.

"I'm so happy you joined us today. It's clear to me you have a particular practice, and you're welcome to come back if you don't mind snagging a corner in the back. It's great to practice in a community, and I'm glad you've chosen this one. People come to class to have me guide practice. It's difficult for me to serve the group if I'm distracted and I was distracted by your practice today."

See, I told you I can be tactful. Sure, it took a few drafts and a couple of run-throughs in front of the mirror.

One of them has become a regular and I haven't seen the other since. It's unfortunate and no matter what you think, I hate to chase people out, but as a teacher, I have to think about the greater service to the class.

I have cobra breathers sometimes. This is a hard one to corral. I talked about the ocean breath in "I AM Breathing, Bitch." A Cobra breather is the client who zealously practices the ujjayi (*ooh-jai*) breath. We're talking pit of vipers. Remember that scene in *Raiders of The Lost Ark* with the snakes? Yeah, that. I've established breathing is a bitch for some people. Moving past the distractions of the external takes practice and moving your attention to the circle of your mat, takes even more. Imagine trying to work out that connection with Darth Vader on the mat next to you. This one I typically cue verbally. "Remember to breathe. Hear the ujjayi in your own ear." Yes, I have to cue consistently throughout the class.

The thing about yoga is the contradiction. Yoga practice is about you. It's about centering your focus on your time on the mat, and letting go of awareness of the ambient distractions. As I've mentioned earlier, one of the niyamas in traditional yoga philosophy is svadhyaya, the examination of the self. We have to dip into Patanjali's *Yoga Sutras* for a bit. The Sutras describe the foundations of the ancient tenets. I've talked about the eight limbs and some of the bigger concepts of what the larger scope of yoga is. Niyamas are the things you DO to move into a higher state of being. Svadhyaya is in part to understand one's self, but also to move past one's ego, or ahamkara (*aha-m-kar-ah*). Ahamkara serves as one of the lenses through which we perceive our experiences. I like to connect this idea to one of *The Four Agreements*. Don't take anything personally. Nine times out of ten, when people are assholes, it has nothing to do with us. Hey, I'm working on it.

Now, the other thing about ego is it's a competitive douchebag. I say it multiple times because people, particularly workout hounds, need to hear it over and over. *Yoga is not a competitive sport.* I know most things in modern society have taken on that edge, but yoga class should not be included in that category. Breathing like Lord Vader may feel like a win over all of us subtle breathers, but it's really about imposing your process on others. *Whoa, hold up, J, you just said not to take shit personally.* I'm not. I'm reminding folks that while yoga is about you, in a group setting, it's also about the community.

In time, folks come to find a balance. It's also a release of competitiveness. I'll say it one more time for the clown car. Yoga is not a competitive sport. I can't tell you how many people are coming from a Go Big or Go Home place. It's a lot and it takes a while to let that inner nag go silent. Eventually, people figure out my class is a mellow neighborly gig. Of course, they may just figure out that their loud breathing irritates their fellow yogis. Either way, most heavy breathers settle down and enjoy the mood.

Another irritation of most teachers are the folks who are temporally challenged. I'm not a Timekeeper Yoga Nazi. Come into my class a little late or leave early. I don't mind as long as you're mindful of the other people in class. You've been there. Comfortable seated position, moving through pratyahara to dharana as the instructor guides you into your balanced breath and focus toward the practice when BAM! the door to the studio slams shut. Someone stomps into class, they kick of their shoes with a thud, and THWAP —slaps their mat to the floor. Or we're all settling into final relaxation or have been in savasana for almost the full ten minutes, and someone rustles, rolls, clomps, all wordlessly announcing their departure from class. Or my personal favorite, someone from outside the studio opens the door and barges in for some special equipment or a yoga mat like our presence is the problem. It's rude. It's disorderly. It kills the Zen.

This is another awareness issue. These people are so oblivious to anything but their own issues and entitlement. I'm going with Shepherd Book on this one. (Any *Firefly* fans?) "There's a very special level of Hell for child molesters and people who talk at the theater." It's the same for people who tromp in or out of yoga class. I can't do much about these folks besides shoot them a wide-eyed, WTF look. You know, it's the visual equivalent of the Uh-Oh you give toddlers when they do something not quite naughty, but naughty enough. I do offer people the out while we are settling into savasana. "If you need to scoot early, this is the perfect time to bail."

One of my long-term regulars leaves class early twice a month to go get a massage. More power to her. She scoots out after our cool down and before savasana. No muss, no fuss.

There's one more subtle taser offense. Fidgeters. Folks who just can't take a full seven- to ten-minute savasana. Nothing is more frustrating than just hitting your Zen to have the person next to you fiddle, wiggle, cough, adjust, or fuss. It's not quite as jarring as the thwapper or stomper. It's slow and creeping like the drip drip drip of a leaky faucet. It's the Italian Water Torture of yoga. Yeah, that's right. I said Italian. An Italian lawyer invented it. Cue lawyer jokes now. (I actually like my lawyer, so there.) It is so faint and inconsistent that you can't get into the space to ignore it. It's like my hubby snoring. You just can't quite tune it out. You can't smother them with a blanket or pillow, or so my hubby claims.

I try to cue these people before we drop into final relaxation. If you wrestle with savasana or lying in one position for any length of time, take seated meditation instead. It's much easier and quieter when you need to squirm. Over time, you may grow more at ease during these silent stretches, thus, moving closer to actually meditating. And you won't irritate your neighbors. Go figure.

Human beings are not yet biologically hardwired to live in the close numbers we do. We're tribal. Operating harmoniously in large numbers is a relatively new development. We can evolve, but it takes time. Our society is a huge experiment in acceptance and tolerance. It's why societies developed taboos, the Golden Rule, and adages like, *If You Don't Have Anything Nice to Say, Come Sit By to Me.* Oops, did I say that aloud? I mean, don't say anything at all. It's commonsense ethics. Grace and kindness, people. Grace and fucking kindness.

Don't talk at the theater. Hang up the phone if you're checking out at the store. Zipper merge, for fuck sake; I don't care if that asshole blew past you to get three cars ahead of you. Tip your wait staff even if they're slow or your food isn't great (it might not be their fault). Leave fair, non-scathing book reviews for authors. And if you are going to be late or need to leave yoga class early, be solicitous of the other people in class.

CHAPTER 13

As Seen On TV

It never fails. If I give a shout out for my yoga classes in any of my other fitness classes praising the virtues of stretch and strength at the same time someone says, "I do yoga. Fifteen minutes with the DVD in my living room. Does that count?" I'd love to say fuck yeah, (you know there's a big, bad BUT coming) BUT remember when I said I'd love my yoga classes to be seventy-five minutes? Yeah, fifteen minutes is a solid post-workout stretch, but honestly, how many of you even do that? I know exactly how much you stretch. Or in this case don't stretch. I've seen it.

In my cycle classes, there are those dogged few who pedal through to the last five minutes of class. They don't see the value of ten minutes of stretching when they can burn twenty more calories or go another half mile. Even in my Fit Fun Flex class—where Flex is in the class title—people still see the last ten minutes of stretching as a perfect time to motor out. It's all good, but you know you're not stretching. It's the same in most of the balls-to-the wall fitness classes that workout hounds love. Five minutes (at most) of cool down and stretching and, more often, ineffective stretching for the energy or exercises of the workout. I get people in yoga who wonder why their backs ache or their knees ache or whatever body part aches at the moment. Strong muscles are great. Strong and long muscles are healthy. So many jokes, heh heh. Fifteen minutes of yoga? You can take a walk in fifteen minutes. You can nurse a glass of wine in fifteen minutes. You CAN. You can empty the dishwasher. Fold a basket of laundry. Have grown-up, long-term couple sex. (Only in the mornings and only on sleep-in days.) Just saying.

But yoga? Let me think about it.

That said, there was a recent study[1] by University of Illinois researchers detailing the benefits to brain function of a twenty-minute yoga practice. Twenty minutes of hatha yoga significantly improved people's speed and accuracy in terms of working memory. I love science-based benefits, so if twenty minutes of yoga works it works. My problem with this concept is that it doesn't take into account the importance of sequencing.

Following Viniyoga philosophy, I typically have a pose in my head, a goal. To arrive at that pose, I sequence the warm-up to target the muscles we are going to use. That means I'm targeting specific muscle groups that we'll need to activate in order to accomplish the targeted pose. Once we've

---

1   Yates, Diana. "A 20-Minute Bout of Yoga Stimulates Brain Function Immediately After." ILLINOIS, 5 June 2013, news.illinois.edu/view/6367/204796.

moved through the flow to that pose, we have to work our way back. Ease muscles, relieve the response to the practice and get into a space for a brief savasana. We're going to talk the importance of sequencing in "Slow Your Roll, Bitches." For now, take U of I's twenty minute suggestion and mull it over. I haven't even tried to build a twenty-minute flow. Remember, my fucking yoga ideal is seventy-five minutes.

I want seventy-five minutes from you so we can spend fifty minutes in the vinyasa. That leaves warm up time, cool down time, and a solid savasana. In my world. Not everything has to be drive-thru speed. Sure, I want fast, global Wi-Fi and direct flights. I'm not a freak. I'm not quite sold on the "do twenty minutes of yoga" thing. As for yoga videos . . . it is a rare occasion I find one with which I can live.

I'm not trashing the yoga video industry. I think DVD yoga, depending on the teacher, the pacing, and the instruction, is perfectly valid. I know of a couple of fairly decent yoga programs. Do I have issues with them? Duh. Hell, I have an entire library of yoga DVDs. Do I use them? Fuck no. You know why? Because I don't have a dedicated, hard floor space to unroll my mat in front of a television. You know why? Because I have three dogs and two cats who think the minute I hit the floor is an automatic invitation to be rubbed against, crawled upon, licked, sniffed, and any number of other animal rituals of bonding they can perform. I don't care how many videos of goat yoga and cat yoga The Beard sends me. It is not yoga. It's goat parkour.

I have a tough enough time running the vacuum and clearing out the flotsam to get my own YouTube videos put together.

I don't typically practice at home because I have two pseudo-adult sons in the basement and a husband. It's always Mom-this or Honey-that. Even if I can hit adho mukha (*ah-doh moo-kah*) svanasana without interruption, you know what I'm going to see? Friggin' dust bunnies. Frankly, if I'm home with quiet time on my hands, I'm writing or cleaning or weeding or walking dogs or some other thing I need to take care of.

Got a spare room with a tile or hardwood floor? Yoga it up. Got a space in front of the television and kennels for the beasties? Yoga it up. Are all of your offspring out of the house? Yoga it up. Got forty minutes or more of time to devote without distraction? Yoga it up.

The thing about yoga class (hell, any fitness class outside of your house) is you're dedicating a couple of hours to your process and well-being. Before I taught yoga, I dragged my carcass into class on Tuesday evenings and Saturday mornings. It was ME time. No one was asking what's for dinner. No one was asking if we had this or that. No one was asking for gas money. I muted my phone and stepped into the ME moment.

You may have already paid a monthly fee to a gym or recreation center. Figure out exactly how many classes or hours you need to workout in order to break that amount down to five dollars an hour. That's the amount I think a fitness class is worth. Call me cheap if you want, but I am happy paying five dollars to drop into a class or a workout. You have to decide what dollar amount you would be satisfied to pay as a drop-in fee. Would you pay that to sleep longer? Hit the snooze and drop that amount into your savings account. Is that amount worth a glass of wine instead of yoga? Hell, last night I found a sub for my class and finished a bottle of rosé, so yeah, sometimes it is.

Each time you think about not going to the gym, ask yourself if you're willing to exchange X amount of dollars for the extra thirty minutes of sleep, or that glass of wine, instead of what you have already paid. I'm not saying don't skip out. I'm saying put that five dollars into your savings account and drink that wine!

"They" say it takes thirty days to establish a workout habit. After a while, you may actually recognize some faces in class and—if you're into that kind of thing (I avoid it at all costs)—you might meet some new people who can help motivate you to come to class. Okay, I did end up doing coffee on Saturdays after yoga with a group of clients. It wasn't torture. Duh, there was coffee.

If you're damned and determined to do an hour or two of yoga at home, and yes, I mean a full and complete sixty minutes, that's fine. Try to find time to drop into a class once a month or so. A good teacher can help you with alignment in a way you won't glean from a video. Once a month in my Vinyasa Flow class, I dedicate time to a particular asana. We work the alignment and corrections as a group. It's always the day I receive the most feedback. They love it. No matter how familiar you are with the asanas, taking time to focus on posture and muscle isolation can sharpen your understanding of a pose. We tend to form habits and rely on muscle memory as we move without conscious thought. Yoga is a fine balance between non-distraction, focused un-focus, and inward contemplation. Like that sentence? Devoting a bit of attention to our placement can reinforce healthy muscle memory and frankly, get our minds off laundry, weeding, or groceries.

My youngest son always shows an interest in yoga until it's actually time to come to my class. "Why can't you teach me at home? Without the crowd?" For all of the reasons I don't practice yoga at home. That's why.

There's also the gooey part. Practicing yoga in a community creates a different mojo than practicing in front of the television. Part of the benefit of yoga, IMO, is the collective investment. Yes, I know I don't like people. It's a conundrum. I am a teacher, writer, and speaker, so clearly, I should like people, but generally I don't. The thing is, however, I really enjoy the assemblage of people in a yoga class.

So yoga on a screen? Whatever. Sure. Go for it. Just be careful to not fall into the trap of recreating a pose or flow exactly; avoid going past your comfort level. Different yoga bodies move in different ways. Remember, this mama's yoga is about healthy alignment and mindful pacing. It's not a race or a competition. Stick with programs offered by yoga people rather than fitness gurus. I don't care what celebrity they train or which network program they headline. Yoga practitioners will more than likely put together solid flows and offer good verbal cues. Mostly.

Drop into a class occasionally for the personal touch and to refresh your understanding of alignment and posture. I'm going to say it over and over, until you're extremely comfortable and confident ignoring imprudent instruction: avoid programs with words in the titles like *power, weight loss, meltdown, sweat,* or *insanity* (personally, fuck anything called insanity—that should be a no brainer).

I say be confident ignoring imprudent instruction because you need to know your body and your alignment before you can work an energetic flow without injury or strain. I have had clients injure themselves because they forgot they know their body better than anyone else. They fell under the spell of mob mentality and pressure from authority to perform in a manner that didn't serve their well-being. Imma say this again because I've heard it takes three times for people to absorb and ingrain information: *A misguided yoga instructor (or fitness instructor) can cause you injury* . . . especially if you're recovering from injury or illness.

Practicing yoga without mindful placement and alignment can cause more harm than good. It's partly ego. Not just on the clients' part, but I've seen it in teachers. Did I tell you about the yoga teacher who hopped on my back while I was in upavistha konasana (*oo-pah-veesh-tah cone-ahs-anna*) (forward folding, seated wide angle)? He's lucky to be alive. Also, he was kind of a tiny guy, so I quickly threw him off. Pushing a client deeper into a pose is a bad, bad thing.

Some of the yoga programs you might access at home won't take a mindful approach. They are aimed at a generally fit and already flexible audience. Some of those programs are designed for the full tilt, I'm-not-happy-working-out-until-I-might-vomit kind of people. I'm not saying don't use them, but work smart. Always think about the feedback your body is giving you and remember, sharp pain is damage.

Once people find out I teach yoga, they delight in regaling me with yoga injury stories. They are defending their avoidance of yoga. Do I think everyone could benefit throughout their lifetime by practicing yoga and Pilates? Fuck yeah. Am I putting on my religious zealot hat and banging down doors to get people into the yoga studio? Uh, no. I don't have to quote statistics here. Google that shit. You'll find oodles of articles by people claiming yoga destroyed their body. It can and does happen when you approach yoga without any kindness toward your body.

I have a client who struggles with back pain. She insists on going to the chiropractor and has basically written off ever riding a bicycle because "I just can't sit that way on a bike." I have a beautiful, therapeutic, low back flow that would change her life, but she won't go for it because she hurt her back once in a yoga class, eons ago. It's a shame, but she's been burned. I'll never get her into one of my yoga classes. Well, maybe now that she's in the book?

Here's my qualitative break down on numbers: at the beginning of every new year, my classes are full—we're talking twenty or thirty people. By mid-February, ten percent of those folks still come faithfully to yoga. (By faithfully, I mean maybe twice a month.) Without deviation, when folks come back to class they say, "Oh man, my body needed this." If you get into the studio twice a month and find a terrific video to practice at home a few times a week, then you're golden. Just be sure to take care of your fucking body. It's the closest, most intimate friend you're ever gonna have.

CHAPTER 14

If the Yoga Mat Fits

Yoga people spend money. Americans spent sixteen-billion-dollars in 2016 on everything you can possibly imagine related to the practice. Imagine what that number is today. For something that requires minimal equipment, there are yoga products galore. It's one of the most common questions I field. Blocks, bolsters, blankets, mats, socks, clothing, towels, straps, the list goes on and on. It really boils down to comfort and cost.

What kind of yoga mat do I need? It depends of what kind of yoga you plan on doing and how often. It could easily be, what's your favorite color? In a pinch, most yoga studios have mats for clients to use. Mats can run anywhere from ten bucks to over one-hundred-dollars. It's a matter of devotion. Being something of a mysophobe, I always recommend investing in your own mat. Start with a ten-buck bargain. You can pick these up at any multi-purpose store. An average yoga mat runs about 24 inches x 68 inches.

Mats come in all kinds of colors and you can get them with groovy designs. Every new mat is slippery. It takes a few uses for them to get dirty and sticky. For these mats, I do recommend using some sort of quick cleaner after each use. I like the kinds that use lavender or tea tree oil, but a studio may have just a basic wipe or spray. If you're using studio mats, a teacher should cue you to wipe down the mat before you roll it up.

Don't soak it. A quick mist and zoom with a towel is plenty.

These basic mats can usually be washed more thoroughly once every couple of months or so. Follow manufacture recommendations. Just be prepared for that shit to take forever to dry. Many a yoga class has found me with my ass wet from a squishy yoga mat. The great thing about a lower end mat is that it's replaceable. It won't hold up to the wear and tear of three or four classes a week, but if you're hitting a class or two a week, you'll be fine for a year or two.

Mats come in a range of thicknesses and lengths. I do get a lot of clients with the poofy pilates mats and I ask them to move to a yoga mat. The fluffy mats slide and promote an awkward angle on your wrists no matter where you place them. I have a pro weight mat because I was tearing up lower end mats. Hey, I teach six or seven hours of yoga a week. I like a 6 mm mat, which is thicker than average, but it isn't soft by any means. My mat also weighs seven pounds. Yes, seven fucking pounds so don't forget you'll be carrying that shit around.

Closed-cell mats tend to be stickier and reversible, and generally (but not always) made of Poly-Vinyl Chloride (PVC). Even if some companies tout non-toxic and 6P-free, many folks believe these mats still release bad for you chemicals. You'll find yoga mats made of jute or hemp, too; both are natural fibers with zero chemicals and are completely eco-friendly. I've never enjoyed using them because they're scratchy. You also need to read deep into the packaging description because many of these mats are hybrids, containing TPE or 'non-toxic' PVC, which are indeed toxic.

Another alternative is a mat made of cork and natural rubber. I've never tried them. People who use cork mats rave about them. They don't slip. They have antimicrobial properties. If you're doing hot yoga—not my fucking cup of anything—people say cork mats are the bomb. Quality cork mats are expensive. I have a regular client, who received a terrific cork mat from his kids for the Yule holiday. It has placement lines for your feet and he loves it. Surgeon General warning: it's heavy as fuck. Heavier than my pro weight mat.

Start basic and then move your way up. I've tried natural rubber mats. I've tried bamboo mats. Since I haven't tried the cork mat, and I'm nowhere near the end of my current mat, the cork will have to wait. I always end up back with a heavy, closed cell PVC mat. That's just me.

If you're into the environment, and I am, concerns about PVC are real. We can't recycle it. We can't burn it. We can't bury it. The thing is, an old yoga mat can come in handy when you're ready to swap it for a new one. In addition to the offspring, we also have three canines and two cats. Nothing works better for pets than a used yoga mat. I cut one to fit under the litter box and voilà! No kitty litter trails to and from the laundry room. I have two mats cut to size for the backseat of my Honda Pilot so when the pups are taking a ride, dog hair is kept off of the interior and there are fewer slide outs during turns. Another pet trick is to cut mats to fit the bottom of the dog kennels. We have one pup that loves regular dog beds and another who chews them into little snippets. A used yoga mat solves that particular issue.

A yoga mat lines the bottom of my pantry where I keep my booze bottles. The hardwood floor was a little slippery. Placing the bottles on the yoga mat keeps everything stable and in place. I've used a yoga mat as drawer liners and the hubby has the leftovers of a mat under some stuff in the garage. I don't know exactly because I try to stay out of there as much as possible. Talking about wood floors, you know all of those cute furniture pads and felt doohickies? Yeah, chop up an old yoga mat to keep things from scratching and slipping.

I know people who use them as camp mats under their sleeping bags and I have a law enforcement client who uses an old yoga mat for his rifle training. Seriously, Google it. I'm sure you'll find more recommendations than I've given here. I think it's a sound investment, especially at the ten-dollar level, to buy your own mat. Even if you don't become a lifelong yogi.

Purchase a mat that will get you through the first three months of yoga. A 2016 Yoga Alliance study[1] says a third of all Americans have tried a yoga class. Consider how much you'd like to invest in something you may rarely or never use. I think ten to fifteen bucks is a fair price for something you might use as cupboard liner down the road. I mean, actual cupboard liner is much more expensive.

Next item worth investing in, is a yoga blanket. Although, once again, it's a germ thing. I used to take the blankets home in batches from the recreation center and wash them because I didn't know when they were being sanitized. Now I just recommend folks get their own. I prefer the large woven, cotton Mexican blankets. They generally run about fifteen to twenty dollars. The tricky part is finding them. You can look online, but be sure you find a heavy weight, cotton blend.

Blankets are all sorts of helpful. They cushion your knees if you have sensitive kneecaps. The only part of my body that needs cushioning are my

---

1   "2016 Yoga in America Study Conducted by Yoga Journal and Yoga Alliance." Yoga Journal, 13 Apr. 2017, www.yogajournal.com/page/yogainamericastudy.

knees. They can bolster your seated position. I sit on mine, placing it just under my sit bones, during any seated work to help my hip placement. I'm sitting on one this minute in my desk chair because I'm short and who has a phone book these days? Use it as a cover up during a full savasana. I also have a few extra that I love taking with me to Red Rocks Amphitheater. They take the bite out of those hard bench seats and serve as a great seat holder. I've also used them to stay warm after a thunderstorm.

Yoga blocks aren't a necessary purchase. Most studios have them and they're just something more to lug around. The blocks help a body access some poses and aids in healthy alignment in other poses. I only have one because the kids gave it to me for Christmas. It's made of cork and weighs about four pounds. The thing I like about mine is it's wider than your average yoga block. It's four inches wide and offers a bit more stability than a foam block, but I probably wouldn't have purchased one on my own.

A yoga strap, however, is great accessory. Some studios have them and some don't. I used to have a stash of men's neckties as extras. Straps offer you longer leverage for all kinds of stretches. I'm crazy tight in the chest and have massive shoulders, so linking my fingers behind my back is just not comfortable. A strap lets me work on those poses that sometimes include linking your hands or wrists. It's called a binding pose and I'm not a big fan because the bind often forces you into a place you might not have the flexibility to perform. Using a strap helps me work an asana without over stretching or feeling frustrated. Straps can also help you in balance poses. Some straps do double duty by keeping your yoga mat rolled in between classes. I have two different contraptions.

Bolsters are great if a studio has them, but unless you're planning on a serious home practice or adventurous sex, I wouldn't invest in one. Hey, I'm not judging, invest away. I like to keep them in the studio because while I currently don't teach a prenatal yoga class, I often have mammas in class and they are a must to get pregos comfortable in savasana. Clients with knee issues or low back issues often find bolsters are helpful, but an extra blanket can do in a pinch.

I see all kinds of yoga bags. Bottomline, a woven strap with slip loops for my mat works. Mine cost about five dollars, and I have a seven-pound mat. It's not tiny. My big, old canvas bag carries my yoga block, a blanket, my strap, extra straps (neckties purchased at Goodwill), mat cleaner, a microfiber rag, a yoga towel, and other sundries. I'm a yoga teacher. Do you need a big fancy bag? Only if you want one. I used to have a super chi chi yoga bag, but I'm over it. Every time I haul that bag around, I think I've got to streamline, but so far, I haven't found another way.

There's no easy or graceful way to carry a yoga mat, unless you go with an over the shoulder, vertical carrier. Essentially a yoga mat condom with straps.

Frankly, I have way too much shit to only use one of those sleek bags. Any other way and you're taking folks out right and left.

Those are the basics. Everything else is icing. If you have temperature issues, you'll find all manner and style of yoga socks. You can even get little eye pillows to block out light during savasana.

As for clothes, jeez, you could drop a small fortune. Any comfortable, loose-fitting clothing will work. I covered this in "Yoga Pants? Oh Hell No," but I don't mind reviewing. You can spend as much or as little as you want on yoga clothing. Nine times out of ten, I end up in pajama bottoms or basic leggings. I'm short. Most yoga pants are too long and trip me up. I have a client who has a great, and apparently, unending supply of super groovy leggings. I admire them, but if a pair of tights costs more than fifteen dollars, I'll pass. I'm all about the bargain.

Yoga tops irritate me. I'm a large breasted woman who wears a medium, but often has to buy a large or extra-large to accommodate las chichis. Ladies, you're feeling me, right? Not feeling feeling me, but you know. Unless I splurge on a high-end yoga brand, which is rarely, I tend to spill a little over regular fitness tops. Most days I just say fuck it, but some days I'm feeling bloated or a little loose in the belly. On those days, I opt for a sports bra with a tank top.

Whatever you feel comfortable in is what will work for you. Men, you might want to invest in some seven- to ten-inch sports briefs for under your shorts. They just keep the gents secure and discrete. Not to say you can't wear a pair of sweatpants. I also have one client who wears his Tae Kwon Do pants. If you can perform a flying side-kick in them, you can practice yoga in them.

I recommend clients dress in layers no matter the season. We'll warm up during a practice and we'll take a rapid cool down during savasana. You want to be able to peel and add as necessary. I don't wear yoga socks, but almost always have a pair of regular old socks to wear during savasana.

In the winter, I sport a beanie and sometimes a scarf. Dude, I friggin hate winter.

I recommend making the smallest investment necessary if you're just dipping a toe into the yoga waters. Consider upgrades later. My rule is, if it starts to go see-through, develops a hole, or loses its stretchy, then—and only then—will I replace it. And remember, your yoga practice is going to be hit or miss. I'm not trying to discourage you. I've taught yoga for almost fifteen years now. Clients come and go. Sometimes they come regularly for two or three years and then something happens . . . a little thing called Life . . . and they drop down to once or twice a month. Any workout routine, yoga in particular, gets dumped when your schedule goes wonky.

If you can put workout clothes to multiple uses, so much the better. I promise, no one is looking at you and thinking about what you're wearing, unless you're showing something we'd prefer not to see. And if you're feeling judged, find another class, find another teacher. Fuck that noise and find your tribe.

CHAPTER 15

Who Let the Dogs Out?

Feet. Feet are one of those things that polarize most people. Let's face it; feet are not the most beckoning of body parts. In my experience, feet desperately need regular attention. And very few people, especially men, take care of their feet. When I taught school, I laid out a monthly stipend to guarantee my feet were suitable for public view. Hello? Yoga teacher.

In my defense, I taught barefoot in my classroom a lot of days. Until parents complained. "Not professional," or some such claptrap. My classroom had two temperatures — polar icecap (pre-climate change) and Mount Etna (we're talking fire and brimstone). I loved me some polar icecap, but twenty-four students in a basement room, hot enough for Hephaestus to do some master work, wasn't fun. Offering my feet some air kept my boiling point (both literally and metaphorically) down.

I don't wear shoes if I can help it. I'm not a member of the Society for Barefoot Living, but I do see the virtue of shucking footwear as often as fucking possible.

Counterpoint, my hubby doesn't walk barefoot in our house. Seriously. He slides his feet into slippers as he gets out of bed and slips them off at the shower. He returns to them post-decontamination and continues until it's shoe time. Granted, his rationalization is we have three dogs, two cats, and two pseudo-adult offspring at home. Even if we didn't, he still wouldn't walk barefoot in our house.

He also won't touch my feet. I can wash them and he won't fucking touch them. P.S. I have pretty feet. It's not like I'm asking him to embrace some loathsome, monstrous tootsies. Let me tell you, the way to your partner's heart is a bomb diggity foot massage. But he's not having any of it.

I digress. Feet. For the most part, yoga calls for bare feet. I know clients who have chronically cold feet. They wear some variation of yoga socks. Some socks have grippy bottoms, some leave your toes bare, and some are just glorified leg warmers that leave your heel and ball of the foot exposed. Maniacs! I just fucking dated myself. (If you don't get it, look it up.) One client has had a couple of toes amputated, so shoes help her balance. Whatever fucking works.

Bare feet allow you a firm base on your mat. Stability is the name of the game. If you haven't already, you're sure to hear the term *grounded* in a yoga class. I guarantee it will be connected in some way to the muladhara chakra, or balancing overactive mind energy, or energy flow of some kind or another. I don't use that bullshit.

I have to consider my crowd. Not many people in my yoga classes at the town recreation center, come to yoga to hear talk of chakras, roots to rise (note we'll talk stupid yoga cues later), or to be of the motherfucking Earth. Mind you, I'm not pooh-poohing being grounded. I have a great respect for the feet and their role, not only in yoga, but in regard to our general health. I just don't use the fucking hoodoo.

First let's talk feet. This little piggy — sorry, I'll be serious. By age fifty, most people will have walked approximately 75,000 miles. I'm not even talking the extra fucking ten thousand steps thing. Like the rest of our body, or maybe worse than the rest of our body, we treat our feet — well, like goddamn feet. Time to gain a little regard for those dogs.

Your feet have more than fifty bones. Twenty-six in each. Fourteen of those make up your toes! Taken as a whole, that's a quarter of all of the bones in your entire fucking carcass. Think about all of those moving parts — did you? All y'all just wiggled your toes. Don't deny it. Okay, now consider over thirty-three joints linking those moving parts. Are you doing some math?

Add to that, a little more than a hundred ligaments, tendons, and muscles that yoke the complex architecture of those dew-beaters. Feel the awe, bitches. Feel it!

Your foot is divided into three areas. The forefoot includes your toes (phalanges) and the metatarsals. The metatarsal bones sit between your phalanges and the cuboid bones. Some of the most common injuries (and most fucking painful) are metatarsal stress fractures. The mid foot is made up of the cuneiform, cuboid, and navicular bones, collectively called the tarsals. These bones form your arch. Or not, resulting in flat feet, or fallen arches, another fucking painful condition that can cause problems all of the way up the skeletal chain. The foot bone is connected to the leg bone.

Actually, it's connected to the heel (calcaneus bone) that supports the talus bone, which is connected to the leg bones. Or to be precise, the tibia and fibula that make up your lower leg. The human foot is one of the more complex anatomical structures in the animal kingdom. Pretty fucking amazing, right?

Breathe it in for a goddamn minute because I'm adding more. The foot has more nerve endings per square centimeter than any other place in your body. Second only to the clitoris. If you're in doubt, think about the last time you fucked up your toes on the corner of the table leg running for the naughty spray to shoot at the barking dogs. I have one word for you . . . fucking Legos. Okay, that's two words.

We need those nerves to give us real time information about how to walk, where we're walking, and our movement relative to the surface on which we're walking. Mobility and equilibrium. Locomotion and balance. Progression and connectedness. Your feet serve as sensory organs. They give you real time feedback as you walk so you don't end up ass over tits. Are you feeling the fucking love?

The problem with this complex and critical structure, is the list of ailments typically associated with high tech gear, except you can't purchase the extra friggin' warrantee coverage. It's like my shopping list. The number of items never ends and something is always added to the bottom. Plantar fasciitis, bunions, heel spurs, flat feet, and metatarsalgia (pain in the ball of the foot), are just the tip of the fucking iceberg.

On average, every day, we exert tons—I'm talking TONS—of foot pounds of force on our poor piggies. That doesn't include runners, hikers, or other athletes who spend thousands of hours employing those bitches. If you've spent any time on your feet, I don't need to tell you how shitty you feel if your feet are aching and exhausted. Tired and sore feet radiate up the calves and into the rest of the body. Hence, the bliss of a foot massage, ahem, oh dear hubby? Feet are the unsung heroes of the fucking body. It's no wonder consumers spend, on average, eight million dollars on running shoes alone. We're all trying to find the perfect fit.

Ladies, and by ladies, I mean ALL of the ladies (Imma Z snap for my diva queens out there), would you like to tally the dollars you spent on shoes in the last year? Or we could divide the number of pairs by the dollar amount? Or we could talk the sublime pair of red-soled heels you found at an insane discount that fucking murder your feet, but hey, anything for fashion. Don't get me wrong, I spent a good portion of my youth in killer heels. Killer being the operative fucking word on so many levels.

And guys, reality check. Women don't buy sexy shoes for you. We buy them because they inspire our fucking kickassedness. Yes, that's a word.

Now? I have a few pairs of heels, but if any shoes hurt my feet, I don't wear them. I mean right out of the box new those shoes must fit without any pinching, squeezing, or rubbing. And I don't walk distance ---any goddamn distance—in heels. I have a pair of flip-flops in summer and a pair of shearling boots for winter that I wear while schlepping my heels in a bag. Even if my dear hubby eschews my feet, I treat them like the fucking champions they are.

Are you digging what I'm laying down about feet?

Okay, let's get back to the mat. Yoga and your feet. If we spend all of that time squishing our toes into shoes and crushing them with walking, running, standing, and any other foot activity, it stands (heh heh) to reason we need to place some mindful focus on our feet while mindfully focusing on our practice. I don't talk grounding, but I do talk stability and placement. If you're in my class, you'll hear me cue awareness of your trotters as "find your feet." Poses start from the fucking mat up. If you're not solid on your feet, you're a hot wobbly mess. There is no falling in my yoga class, unless it's me and then you can laugh. If I don't get up in about five minutes, call 911. Laugh first, fucking 911 second.

"Find your feet" means take your time. Make any adjustments in or out so you feel stable on the mat. And yes, I do say all of that at one point or another during class. I also tell clients to lift up their toes and spread them out. This is more effective instruction than "ground yourself" because it helps clients feel the full surface of their foot on the fucking mat. (Plus, people interpret things they hear differently.) You think the game Telephone was tough because you whispered? I'll come back to this in "Stupid Shit Yoga Teachers Say."

With several poses, finding the feet is a no-brainer, especially when the teacher says the thing that finally clicks in your brain. No matter what, clients are surprised to have fatigued feet at the end of practice. It's primarily because their feet have remained grounded. Yes, I fucking used it. The thing is, we don't use our feet on a regular basis the way we use them in a yoga practice.

Yoga is great for all kinds of foot maladies—not a full-blown cure—but solid treatment.

Stretching cramped feet can improve blood circulation. I'm pretty sure by now you understand that improved blood flow is fucking good for your pieces and parts. Opening up space in your feet relieves pinching and scrunching of those nerve endings I mentioned. Spreading your toes strengthens the hundred muscles and tendons that articulate your toesey woseys and help relieve bunions, hammer toes, and fallen arches. Good foot placement improves your overall posture from the fucking ground up (heh heh, I'm on a roll). Better posture often addresses some types of back pain, knee pain, hip pain, oh hell, all kinds of structural-related pain.

Treating your feet with respect can be an overall boon to your fucking health. Foot cramps are often a sign of dehydration or mineral deficiencies. Physical symptoms of diabetes often show up first in your feet and legs. Chronic burning and swelling in your feet and toes could indicate gout. There's nothing more irritating than nerve numbness in our feet, except nerve numbness in our fucking hands. That crazy, crawling ant sensation can be a pinched nerve or nerve damage from wearing those goddamn stilettos.

And to be completely superficial, offer your fucking feet some beauty care before a yoga class, because I do sometimes have to touch peoples' feet. Give them a regular scrub. Trim your friggin' toenails. Go barefoot occasionally to air them out. Smelly feet come from shoes and socks. Don't wear the same pair of socks two days in a row, if you can help it. Rotate shoes and allow them fresh air. Now, about fifteen percent of the population has exceptionally sweaty, stinky feet. (Hey, Offspring, did I mention I love you?!) This comes from a bacterium called Kyetococcus sedentarius. Give a zinc-based foot powder a try to keep your feet dry.

If eyes are the windows to the soul, then your feet are the gateways to, I don't fucking know, but they do say something about you and it would probably be best if it wasn't, "OMG! Put those fucking dogs away!"

CHAPTER 16

Baby Got Back. Cervical. Thoracic. Lumbar.

Nine times out of ten, it's back pain that drives clients to my yoga classes. Approximately thirty million Americans experience an aching back at any given moment. Worldwide, back pain has been labeled the leading cause of disability. In fact, even now, as I'm sitting at my desk working on this chapter, my low back is fucking killing me. I make no secret of my office chair issues. I used to sit on a balance ball chair in my classroom, but you teachers out there know how much time you spend sitting. I split my time between standing and my balance ball.

Recent medical studies have shown1 that yoga is twice as effective in relieving back pain as most other exercises. Sadly, a wide and colorful variety of opioids are prescribed for over forty percent of back pain cases. Hmm, I could descend into a tirade on the opioid crisis in America along with our dependence on prescription drugs, but that's for someone else to write.

Also, it must be noted that some back conditions and injuries can be worsened with yoga practice. Part of this has to do with the type of damage sustained, and I'm going to go out on my limb to say part of this can be exasperated by a weak instructor . . . and by weak, I do mean stupid as fuck. I don't mean literally stupid, although it could be the case in some instances. I mean yoga stupid. It's one of the things I love about Viniyoga. Yes, I'm going to go on about Vini-fucking-yoga . . . AGAIN.

Viniyoga is all about the health of the spine. Psst, that's your back we're talking about. The variations of the postures, the sequencing of the flows, the intense breathing component all work to support and nurture your spine. Can you dig it? Since most of the clients I work with couldn't tell lumbar vertebrae from cervical vertebrae, including some of the clients who have had a spinal fusion, we need to start with the basics. Baby's got one.

Welcome to Julia's lecture on Your Spine. Cue the silly animated documentary music. The vertebral column is important. Duh, it serves as the conduit for your spinal cord. Last time I checked that was a critical piece of operations. The brain and the spinal cord make up your central nervous system. In that big ol' noggin of yours, your brain is made up of billions of neurons that generate electrical and chemical impulses across junctions called synapses. Those impulses travel across synapses and continue on to your spinal cord where they get distributed from your central nervous system (brain and spinal cord) to your peripheral nervous system that branches out to the rest of your body. These include blinking, breathing, stretching, digesting, and all of the other responses to external stimulation.

Different areas of the spinal cord relay communication to various regions of the body. Consider it the major trunk line, wait — am I dating myself? Shit, how many of you still have a landline? Let's back this thing up. The spinal cord is the main thoroughfare for information, and that information is redirected further down the chain through the sensory-somatic and autonomic nervous systems. Are you still with me? And information travels in both directions along these routes. Given the amazing complexity of the body, information can easily become waylaid in places.

If you're a side sleeper like me, you frequently impinge the radial nerve, which runs down, between your Pectoralis Minor, Pectoralis Major, Supraspinatus, and Subscapularis muscles. The shoulder is a complex joint. I'll discuss shoulders in more detail in book two on poses. Stay tuned! Sliding down through all of these muscles, the radial nerve can get pinched. Welcome to the nightmare of hand-tingling numbness. Another reason my radial nerve gets hitched up, is that I'm not a delicate flower. I may have mentioned I have the shoulders of a linebacker. This heavier muscle structure serves me well in most instances, but when I work my upper body without an effective stretch afterward, my radial nerve definitely complains about the crowding. You see how important your nervous system is?

Your spine, divided into regions around your spinal cord, is made up of thirty-three individual bones, though only the top twenty-four are designed to move. The cervical spine consists of the vertebrae in your neck (C1 through C7 vertebrae). This section of the spinal cord is responsible for controlling the neck muscles, diaphragm (an important part of your breathing muscles), wrists, triceps, and fingers.

Next down the line is the Thoracic spine (T1 through L2). This region of the spinal cord deals with hands, trunk (intercostals and the abdominals), and ejaculation. Yep, I said it. Because men experience more spinal cord injuries than women at a ratio of four to one, the research naturally has a gender bias, so it's hard to quantify the effects on women's sexual health. I'm happy to enter into a debate about gender bias and feminism in the medical sciences, but that is also an entirely different book. Wow, who knew this chapter would be loaded with anti-patriarchal rants? Back to your back.

The Lumbar spine contains the L2 through the S1 vertebrae and protects the nerve roots for the hips, quadriceps, hamstrings, and feet. Technically, the spinal cord doesn't run through the Lumbar spine. It stops in the lower Thoracic and splits off like distributaries from a river. The Lumbar spine does the lion share of weight bearing for the spine. Because of this branching out of the nerves, spinal cord injuries rarely happen in the Lumbar region, but with it being the workhorse of the spine, it's where I see the most common issues in clients.

The lumbar spine is crazy interconnected with your hip joints. You have the Erector Spinae muscles holding you upright, and also affecting the lumbar region is the Intersegmental muscle group, the Quadratus Lumborum, and the Multifidus. On the superior side, you've got the hip flexors going which include the Iliopsoas bundle. As if that isn't enough moving equipment, we're also dealing with tension and forces from the abdominals, and I haven't even started on the Gluteus Maximus or the other muscles in the legs. It's no wonder lower back pain affects over three million people per year in the United States alone. Those numbers only include people who have sought medical treatment.

What the fuck does all of this mean? It means that lower back pain can be caused by a shit ton (yes, that is a scientific measurement) of factors. Most of those factors can be counteracted by some simple stretching and as that is the case, think of what an hour of yoga practice can do.

Remember "Yoga Ain't for Sissies"? I only hinted at what improving your core strength and stability could do. There's a little thing called the lumbar-pelvic rhythm. This rhythm is the ratio between flattening the lumbar curve and stretching it (tucking your tailbone or dropping it like it's hot). Low back pain is often the result of mechanical disproportion in standard lumbar-pelvic stability. That was a big sentence. Let me sum up: any position—no matter how slight—outside of normal in your lumbar spine, can cause aches and pains.

In people with tight hamstrings, the hammies tug down on your Ischial tuberosity (remember those sit bones?) rotating your pelvic cradle down toward the floor. This causes low back pain. For me, particularly after cycle classes, my deep lateral hip rotators (Piriformis and Quadrates femoris) get super tight and tug outward on my pelvic cradle creating all kinds of nasty ache in my lower back. If you have tight adductors, along with the other muscles of the inner thigh (the bane of my existence is a not so little muscle called the Sartorius), that can tug forward on your pelvic cradle resulting in — all together now — lower back pain!

Yoga gets me through teaching five or six fitness classes a week.

Now to be fair, there isn't enough yoga for some of these muscles, and that's where my intimate relationship with Mr. Foam Roller comes into play. Again, another book, although I have been known to bust out the foam rollers when I have a smaller class. It ain't pretty, but you'll feel fabulous an hour later. I also highly recommend finding a talented massage therapist who can do some serious deep tissue work. There isn't anything gooey about deep tissue work, but it can relieve soft tissue issues when stretching can't.

Balancing the forces between your abdominal core and your lumbar spine takes time and patience. I tell my clients that strong abdominal muscles help support their lower backs. Here are my rough guidelines to identifying the type of back pain and the recommended adjustment. Any sharp pain is typically a warning of potential damage. We need to adjust what you're doing or actual damage might happen. Ache (nothing sharp) from just above your waistband down to your tailbone, is muscle pain. (I'm talking about a waistband sitting where a waistband is supposed to. None of this pants-slung-around-your-hips bullshit. Think Mom jeans.) Ache in this area after yoga or pilates means we've worked your core and the structure of your lumbar is feeling the results.

Ache above that means we've worked the core and back muscles, possibly chest. Strengthening these structures improves our overall posture and takes some of the weight off of the lumbar spine, thus, improving the balance of our lumbar-pelvic rhythm. (Go ahead, I'm doing it. I'm humming a few bars of "Walking in Rhythm.")

Lengthening and strengthening the muscles that support the spine helps us fight gravity, and I'm repeating myself, but we all know what an asshole gravity can be. Remember, you don't actually shrink with age, not significantly. Our core and back strength weakens, and we slouch. Now there are all sorts of little gadgets cropping up to remind you to sit up straight, but do you really think they'll be less annoying than your mother or grandmother?

Another little tidbit . . . back surgery sucks. A National Institutes of Health study[2] reported that less than five percent of folks with chronic back pain need surgery. The more terrifying statistic is that almost forty percent of those surgeries fail, requiring more surgery.

We're so used to instant results that a lot of my clients grow frustrated with the baby steps. Recovering from an injury, particularly back injuries, takes a lot of time. As I said earlier, it's taken time to get our bodies in their current state, and a back injury can a be a sudden indicator we weren't treating our body well in those years. It can be debilitating.

Okay, so for some of you that train may have already departed the station. BUT, (oh waffles and tarantulas, surely you know by now there is always a but) here's the thing about Viniyoga and The F*cking Yoga Company: there is a mad variety of yoga poses to help stabilize your back without twisting or bending. A Viniyoga instructor or a certified yoga therapist, or even a conscientious yoga instructor with common sense, can help modify poses for you.

First, always do everything your physical therapist and surgeon recommend. If you've got approval to take a yoga class, always go early and have an honest conversation with the instructor. Look for classes labeled

2   Baber, Zafeer, and Michael A Erdek. "Failed Back Surgery Syndrome: Current Perspectives." Journal of Pain Research, Dove Medical Press, 7 Nov. 2016, www.ncbi.nlm.nih.gov/pmc/articles/PMC5106227/.

"gentle" or "therapeutic," because true Viniyoga classes are hard to find. Even a beginning yoga class could serve if the instructor is aware of your limitations and willing to offer modifications. If that isn't the case, get the fuck out of there.

Repeat after me: baby steps.

If you're in the group who fortunately missed the back injury train, get off your duff and move. Walk. No running around the pool. Walk to a yoga class and offer your body some sincere grace and kindness. If you punish it regularly, you better be giving it some love. Cuz fuck if it won't make you pay.

CHAPTER 17

Zen And the Art of Chocolate Cake
(Caution: Hoodoo Ahead)

The only thing you're going to be comfortable doing in yoga class is being uncomfortable. That's one of the processes of yoga. When I use terms like *fun*, *comfortable*, or *strong* they are relative to the context of fucking *discomfort*.

"You keep using that word. I do not think it means what you think it means." — Inigo Montoya

Letting go of the discomfort to find unity between the breath, body, and mind is the next process of yoga. This is the Zen I've been talking about. I could quantify it as the Holy Fuck of Zen, but some would doubt the Zen of a statement like that. Fuck 'em if they can't take a joke.

When I'm guiding a vinyasa, sometimes we move into modified ardha parsvottanasana (*are-dah parsh-voh-tahn-ahs-anah*) (half forward folding pyramid). I cue a soft bend in both knees. I call it the squish. A soft bend means no hyperextension (locking of the knees); you are totally into the hamstring, no cheating. In this position, a whole lot is going on with the body. The quadriceps are firing. The gluteus maximus are firing. I cue a squared position of the hips and drawing the front of the hip away from the extended ankle. The transverse abdominal is firing. Both the internal and external oblique abdominals are firing. Like I fucking said, a lot is going on. I know when a class has discovered all of these muscles working together to make this pose heat up; it's a collective Holy Shit moment. The energy of the room shifts. People often let out oomphs or humphs. I usually respond with, "Say hello to your hamstrings for the first time today, or maybe the first time ever." I can call this discovery a lot of things; anxiety, unease, energy, or heat, but it all amounts to the same thing: fucking uncomfortable. There is a fine line between discomfort and outright pain. Remember, this is a step back from cowboy up.

That holy shit feeling? It's change. And I don't have to tell you how much friggin' disquietude that change causes most people. This is the process of yoga, even in the discussion of yoga equals physical practice. My brand of fucking yoga encompasses mind, body, and breath even if I'm not blatantly referencing the Sutras. It's the letting go of the discomfort that allows our bodies to move past it. You take a deep breath and let the brain go mushy. I know this sounds a lot like the drill sergeant bitch's order to disconnect your body from your mind, but it's really about working together to go somewhere different. It's not disjointed separation. It's connection, union, and trust experiencing the fucking unease as a complete entity. It's as one of my favorite authors, Natalie Goldberg, describes in writing, "It is a great moment passing through you." And not thinking about chocolate cake. Seriously, you thought I was going to leave it all airy fairy? The thought of chocolate cake or a terrific margarita can fuck up that mind mush faster than you can say mind mush.

These moments in class are the exact moments when your brain and body start freaking the fuck out. In ardha parsvottanasana, muscle memory might demand you hyper extend your knee to take up the discomfort your hamstring is feeling at both stretching and strengthening at the same fucking time. Your hamstring says, "Goddamn it, Knee! It's your job to lock so I don't have to work this hard." Your knee replies, "Fuck you, Hammie. It's about time you did your fair share." Your brain is moaning, "Holy ghost and tulips! Whose idea was this fucking yoga thing? I think we'd rather be sipping a margarita." That's the physical challenge of yoga. It's mental chatter. The noise is a defense mechanism, a distraction from being in the moment in union. Goddamned restful activity.

It's exactly the time when your brain wonders if you fed the dogs, or left lunch money out for the offspring. Or thinks you're out of your friggin' mind for doing this. The brain is an egomaniac. It likes to be the focus of our attention. To be quiet, even for an hour of yoga class is fucking torture.

It's a tenacious three-year-old chanting, "Look at me. See me? Look at me! Look what I can do." And thoughts of chocolate cake or Mezcal—two things I fucking love vie for my attention.

The Zen comes from moving past the chatter. We aren't ignoring the sensations of our physical discomfort. We're acknowledging it. We fucking honor it. Then we move past it with acceptance. It's another means to move into pratyahara (detachment from the external to move our attention inward) and then dharana (concentration, focus on the nuances of the energy, the process of breath) and finally into dhyana (the state of being keenly aware without focus). That's fucking yoga, bitches!

That is why so many practitioners of yoga resist the western concepts of Hatha yoga (hatha in this context being the purely physical practice). You cannot move through this process in a class that impels you to change poses with every inhale and exhale. It's too fast. Speed removes the intent of the asanas. When the pace moves too quickly, you lose any quiet space in which you can occupy. You can't move through this process if the instructor is shouting at you. It's too loud. You can't move through this process if the instructor is talking the entire time. It's too fucking annoying.

My goal is to get you into your fucking skin and rejoice. Okay, rejoice might be too strong of a word. How about not grimace? It's a place to start.

No, I don't talk about the eight-limbed path. Some of the philosophy of yoga and Buddhism and Hinduism—and let's face it, Islam and Christianity—has grown off-putting in this mass marketing, commercial business of fucking spirituality. Add metaphysics, astrology, parapsychology, and all of the other hoodoo competing for airtime and your hard-earned dollars . . . it's a lot of shit to sort through, let alone digest.

I'm going to step into the fucking whoohoo of yoga for a minute. Even if you're not practicing the whole kit and caboodle, you can find an hour of silence. Not actual silence because you're in a room with a lot of other people, but when those people concentrate on a common goal there is a generation of energy. The fucking vibe. Yes, I said it. In a yoga class or in church or at a great concert, the vibe is gooey and benevolent. Moving, feeling, thinking in unison (as close to it as possible) and repetition becomes a friggin' meditation.

Somewhere in the community of the class, you let go of everything, and you mellow into a place unperturbed by the small shit. You fucking Zen out. All of the wheels are turning, all of the cogs are meshing, and all of the tumblers click. When I hit this in class, I'm sure to skip a pose in the pattern we've been working. Unless chocolate cake intrudes. The one time I fell in class chocolate cake was the culprit, and it proceeded to take out the rest of class as well in a fit of giggles, but that was cathartic in its own fucking right.

This is why the ceremony and gathering at churches and other holy places is such a refreshing, fucking high. It's the altruistic side of mob mentality and it's a seriously groovy thing. When you wade deeper into the waters of the yoga pool and move toward the eight-limbed path, the reverberation is maintaining that gooey fucking benevolence for more than just an hour.

One of my clients regularly comes to my Last One to Bed Is A Rotten Egg yoga class. It's on a Tuesday night at seven-thirty. Some nights it's a fucking challenge for me to show up because the large glass of wine sure is tempting, especially in the depths of goddamn winter. This client brings her kids to the recreation center with her. They swim or play basketball or sit outside of the studio and work on homework. Okay, they could be playing video games or something, but you know what I mean.

I'm pretty sure they have strict "You may die" orders not to interrupt yoga class for any petty sibling bullshit. Hey, I have three kids, I know what goes on between siblings. The minute I open the door after the full ten-minute savasana, one of her kids rushes in to have first contact. I'm guessing to mitigate whatever situation arose while my client attended class.

Every time, every single time, she puts her hand up and calmly says, "In a minute, outside." She moves with deliberation to get her shoes on and gather her things. All the while her offspring are hopping from one foot to the other, impatient to get on with the rest of the evening. She is holding onto the Zen zone and more fucking power to her.

Here's the thing, even if it's not yoga, devoting time to any kind of exercise without interruption or intrusion can really clear out the cobwebs. I know a lot of folks feel they have to distract their brain from the discomfort of whatever the workout that day might be. The myth of diversion in exercise is that you'll actually work out if you're not so fucking miserable. I'm talking about that bank of televisions in front of the treadmills tuned to HGTV. Think about distractions in your work environment or the minute you take a phone call and your kids sense you're unavailable. Mine are in their twenties and they still innately know when I'm on the fucking phone. It takes an average of thirty minutes to recover focus from an interruption. Thirty minutes to regain your center and find your fucking flow again.

The concept of distraction doesn't apply to laundry. Distract the shit out of folding laundry.

Remember, I said yoga is about being in your body. Reconnecting with your physical quality. Any workout should be the same. The one exception to this, proven by psychologists[1] (it is too a science), is music. A great playlist can optimize the efficacy of your workout.

---

1   Thakare, Avinash E, et al. "Effect of Music Tempo on Exercise Performance and Heart Rate among Young Adults." *International Journal of Physiology, Pathophysiology and Pharmacology*, US National Library of Medicine, 15 Apr. 2017, www.ncbi.nlm.nih.gov/pmc/articles/PMC5435671/.

Sure, I have a collection of wooey new age music same as any other yoga teacher and I use it in my therapeutic classes. Don't tell me people can't find the Zen to rock music. The fuck you say. I pride myself on my playlists, even going so far as to tailor them for specific clients. I have a Guitar Hero yoga playlist for one of my regular clients (Shout out to Randy!), featuring a lot of heavy guitar riff bands from the seventies. Even if you're on the treadmill or walking outside, stick with the earbuds or total silence. Avoid grabbing a magazine or watching whatever is on the gym television. Be in your fucking body for a bit. See what you discover, even if it might be "OMG, when is this hour going to be over?"

Remember how great you'll feel after a shower and a glass of something!

Personally, I dig the current Dali Lama. Ya gotta love a man who tweets with the same smiling compassion he offers the groups to whom he speaks. You have to check him out. Yes, he's THE Buddhist monk, but his wisdom is super down to earth. Plus, he's a fucking giggler. Who doesn't love a giggler? I also adore Thich Nhat Hanh (*tic knot han*). Another super down to earth guy who grins from ear to ear. Seriously, I've never seen the man not grinning. And you know those guys are not doing shots of Mezcal, at least I'm pretty sure they aren't.

Thich Nhat Hanh said, "People have a hard time letting go of their suffering. Out of the fear of the unknown, they prefer suffering that is familiar." I've spent part of a lifetime with people who live this way. Clinging to whatever drama or illness or trouble they can rather than move into a different space. This is the bigger life size version of the Holy fuck of Zen I'm talking about.

Step onto the mat, be out of your life for an hour, and fucking embrace the body you have in this moment. In the process, you will move past the moment and into a healthier body, a healthier state of mind, and then go devour that piece of chocolate cake with joy and without fucking regret. Chocolate cake works for wrinkles same as Botox any day and is a lot cheaper.

CHAPTER 18

Mumbo Jumbo or Stupid Shit Yoga Teachers Say

To be fair, yoga and Pilates are tough to teach. The whole get-in-touch-with-your-body thing is fucking hard. I just spent fifteen minutes after a yoga class with a client trying to help him relax his lower body in sukhasana (*soo-kahs-uh-nuh*), which is easy seated pose. Didn't realize there was an easy seated pose, did you? Think crisscross applesauce without stacking your legs. It may be hard to access if you are tight in the hips. This client is a swimmer. Very tight in the hips.

Frankly, as Americans we've spent a good portion of our time ignoring our bodies. It's a leftover from those whacky, witch-burning Puritans. The learning curve in both yoga and Pilates is off the fucking charts. You think learning to work your new phone is tough? Let's play a little game.

Are you sitting? Okay, sit up straight and place your feet on the floor. Look at your legs. Are they lined up with the center of your hips? Touch the iliac spine. Those low and forward hipbones, not the iliac crests, which are high and out to the side. Line your femurs up with where your hands are. And then move your feet to ninety degrees. Activate the lower portion of your transverse abdominis and your obliques. That's your low belly, FYI. Now, take your focus into your thighs. Are they fucking tense? Relax your legs all of the way down to your feet. Did you go back to slouching a little? See? It's harder than you think. Remember, ninety percent of how we use our bodies comes from fucking habit.

Not all habits are bad. We develop habits to move through our routines more quickly and effectively. Let's face it, there are hundreds of little things during the day that don't require our direct focus. It's also a matter of the function of the brain. Neurons are the basic working units in the brain. They transmit information through the nervous system to other parts of the body. When a group of neurons fire together in response to certain input, they build connections to each other. Fucking efficiency. This is why when you forget the reason you walked into a room, okay, this might just be me, but when I fucking forget why I walked into a room, it helps to leave and retrace my steps. I'm triggering those neurons to fire in sequence again so I can remember what the fuck I was doing.

Over time and with the same sensory input, those connections get stronger. They become habits. It how our brain works on autopilot. We fucking program it. It really is an amazing process. And no, I never get tired of saying it. Playing an instrument. Learning to type (a long time ago, in a land far away, we had these machines called typewriters. And when some of us were riding fucking dinosaurs to school, we had to learn to type automatically). Swimming. Driving a stick shift. (No fucking dinosaur references, it's a life skill okay?) All of those things we file away in our brain and never have to think about doing, are neatly programmed.

Yoga and Pilates are physical activities designed to break those connections.

I can verbalize, guide you to visualize, and physically correct yoga poses a million fucking times, but until you discover the feeling of engaging your core and lengthening your spine, it's moot. It's a bloody challenge that isn't limited to one type of client. Men, women, young, old, we all hear things differently and what works for one person may not translate for another. Yoga is a physically internal process and we're wrestling autopilot every inch of the fucking way. Of course, instructors use all kinds of metaphors and verbal cues to get you to feel your body and its different placements. Yes, some of them are fucking hooey.

One of my regular clients, Charlie, has been coming to three or four yoga classes a week and my cycle classes. He said this week, "You know, you say things over and over and until today, I couldn't feel what you were talking about. Today, it all finally clicked and BAM! I felt like I was doing yoga."

In defense of yoga teachers, we're trying to get you to understand the individual movements your body is capable of and sometimes that manifests by any fucking means necessary. Okay, it doesn't mean that, but we're trying.

In no particular order, here are some phrases yoga teachers use, a few I'm guilty of, a few absolutely confuse, and a few that are absolute bullshit. I've taken an ibuprofen to ease the strain of eye roll and now that I think about it, maybe I should put this chapter off until I've had a couple of glasses of wine. Or mayhap a gummy. Fuck it, here we go.

Soften your ribs

What the fuck does this mean? Soften my ribs. It's impossible to soften your ribs. Not only is this impossible, it runs into the realm of disbelief. A technically minded client is tagging this as unmitigated bullshit and you've lost them.

I know what this cue is trying to accomplish. All right, sit up. Take a deep breath. Fill your lungs so you expand your chest and ribcage. Feel that stretch? Okay, now cough. Cough again. Feel the contraction of your ribs? They squeeze and drop down. This is some fucking core work. I like to use the phrase *anchor your ribs*, but only after the cough exercise. Anchoring your ribs activates your transverse abdominis, rectus abdominis, and the muscles between the ribs called the intercostals. More fucking power to the core.

Root to rise

This is some serious waddle twaddle with no real meaning. Root to rise can encompass intention of the practice with fucking metaphors for how the practice will represent your life. In my opinion, not falling is a terrific intention. Just saying. The root to rise thing can reference the foundation of the pose whether a teacher is talking about your feet or your hands. Stupid. This is also a cue for being grounded in a pose.

The only poses it makes sense to reference grounding are the standing poses. I like to use the phrase *find your feet*. This is equally bullshit because, duh, they're at the end of my fucking legs. I cue this after a reminder about feeling the full surface of your foot on the mat. Let's work this together. Put your feet on the floor. Now, lift and spread your toes and then press evenly down with your entire foot. That's fucking finding your feet. I also use this to prompt folks take their time to find their balance. If you have secure foot placement, you are unlikely to be off kilter when you move into the full expression of a pose. Weebles wobble[1]. People fucking fall.

Enmesh your feet

This just sounds silly. First, who in a yoga class (besides vocabulary nerds) is thinking like a fucking thesaurus? I love words more than most. I'm a

---

1   This is a call back to a toy line by Hasbro Playskool called Weebles. They were egg-shaped, bottom-heavy roly-poly golems of people and animals that wobbled, but didn't fall down. Maybe my spiritual representation?

former Literature/English teacher. Of course I know what enmesh means. A lot of people probably do as well, but in yoga class? Fuck that. Enmesh is not a good synonym for anything to do with feet unless you're being hunted with a bola or a snare net. Think about this; can you embroil your feet in a nefarious plot? Don't be a smart ass. Of course, you can't.

This is a bullshit instruction to anchor your feet. See the above paragraph and my use of *find your feet*.

Wring out your liver

Hell for breakfast! This falls under the well-worn category of friggin' hogswallop. You can't wring out any of your internal organs. You don't release fucking toxins. You can't massage your internal organs. Okay, I did once have a Mayan Arvigo Abdominal massage, but it's best forgotten. Bleh. You can squeeze organs by twisting, but it doesn't create any detoxification or improved function. Go back and revisit "Did that Bitch just Fart?" This is gobbledy gook used by instructors who haven't a fundamental understanding of how human biology works. Fucking science, people!

I like to explain effective twisting by starting with a geographical reference. You have a belly button, right? (Okay, honorary daughter, you might not and thinking about it just freaks me the fuck out. Love you!) I'm going to direct the conversation to the mostly holy Gary Kraftsow, who was one of the first American yoga teachers to be certified by TKV Desikachar. I say mostly because I disagree with some of his stuff (you are NOT surprised, are you?) In Viniyoga, the primary intention of twisting is to lengthen and rotate the spine[2]. It has nothing whatsoever to do with wringing out your fucking liver.

Twisting starts with the belly button because that's the center of your core. Sit up straight and take a deep breath. As you exhale, start your twist behind your belly button rather than your shoulders. This is more fucking core work. I don't know about you, but I can't feel my liver nor could I point it out to you on a map. I do, however, know exactly where my belly button is.

Straighten your elbows or your knees.

This one on the surface seems straight forward, heh heh heh. This falls into the "don't fucking do it" category. If I could prevent everyone in any of my fitness classes from hyperextending or straightening their arms I would. It serves no good purpose and causes problems with your wrists and up the chain to your arms and shoulders, especially when you're lifting weights.

Same goes for knees. In fact, I say the exact opposite 99.9% of the time. I tell clients to soften their knees and elbows. If I'm slipping into fucking Nazi mode, I will say, "bend your elbows," but that prompts a deeper angle than I'm looking for from clients. If your elbows or knees are soft in a weight-bearing pose, then your muscles are doing the work rather than your joints. Joints move. Muscles support and work.

---

2   Kraftsow, Gary. *Yoga for Wellness: Healing with the Timeless Teachings of Viniyoga.* Penguin/Arkana, 1999.

Straighten your hair. Straighten your spine. Straighten out your spice cabinet, but not your fucking elbows or knees.

Tuck your tailbone

I am absolutely guilty of using this one. I think tilting your pelvis is more physically accurate, but people go weird when I say pelvic-anything. I blame Elvis. Tucking your tailbone means rocking your hips slightly forward. This results in lengthening your lumbar curve, stretching your lower Erector Spinae muscles, the Quadratus Lumborum, and the lower connections of the Latissimus Dorsi. It also involves activating your lower abdominals. Four for the fucking price of one. Such a small movement, but it packs a punch. So tuck away.

Stuck between two panes of glass

Oy, so many fucking problems with this one. This lovely phrase is typically used in trikonasana (*tree-kone-aa-sun-aa*) or triangle pose. First, everyone pushes this pose past their limits, so the suggestion should have less to do with glass and more to do with the approach. Second, very few people have the alignment flexibility to get their body flat in this pose. It's bullshit. (Yes, I sing-songed that a little.)

I'm more concerned with people's fucking knees in this pose because there is a strong tendency to lock them. (Hyperextension equals bad.) They also swing their extended arm behind their bodies to mimic the feeling of the rotation of the torso needed for this *two panes of glass* nonsense. That isn't good for the shoulder girdle. A good way to work this pose is to stand against a wall. Extend your arms and tick tock like a clock into your lateral bend. I guarantee you'll have to stop somewhere around your knee, or you will peel off of the fucking wall.

That's lateral extension and healthy alignment.

Ears inline with your biceps.

This is a terrible instruction. It often results in people shrugging their shoulders up toward their ears. Relax your fucking shoulders! You're going to hear that a lot in the next book, so buckle up. This prompt is frequently given during adho mukha svanasana (downward facing dog). I have so many objections to this idea and frankly, all of the instructions for downward facing dog that I've devoted an entire chapter to it in my book on poses.

In no pose, ever, should you fucking align your biceps with your ears. Oh shit, maybe a couple, but they involve lying on your back or taking lateral extension. Shit, this one is complicated.

Don't align your biceps with your ears in downward facing dog, ever.

Listen to Your Body

I like this one, no really, and I use it frequently. If you haven't picked up my vibe that yoga is all about developing an intimate relationship with your body by now, I don't know what you've been reading this whole time. Listen to your body and it will provide you with immediate fucking feedback. Pain is the signal that you are doing damage. Discomfort is a sign you are making change. Part of the process of yoga is learning the difference between the two.

Hey, if your body is unhappy, focus your awareness on the why. If it's pain, back off of a pose. If it's anxiety or agitation, try to figure out the source. Concentrate on your breathing and dig deeper. It could be mental, emotional, or physical. Balancing poses are a great indicator of mental noise. A lot of clients think if they're struggling with a balancing pose it's because of poor balance. Nope, it's more often they are letting the chit chat in their brain get the better of their practice. Listen. To. Your. Fucking. Body.

Hip openers

Bullocks. Bonk. Hokum. Hooey. Your hips don't fucking open. Okay, if you're very pregnant and close to delivering a baby, your hips will spread a bit to make room for that newbie noggin. And THEY WILL NEVER FUCKING GO BACK. I may be harboring a smidge of bitterness on this score. In every other instance, your hips don't open. You can stretch your hip flexors, a bundle of muscles known as the iliopsoas. You can stretch the muscles of the hip girdle and rotators, though these are not fun stretches, and it takes a little doing to reach the muscles. I have a close and personal friend called Mr. Foam Roller that I almost like better than my hubby. Almost. You can stretch the muscles of your inner thigh (Sartorious and the Gracilis); they help your flexors, but they are a bitch to stretch.

We can and do stretch all of those muscles. We do not open our fucking hips. We can open our eyes. We can open our minds. We can open our arms and yes, we can open our legs, but that's a whole different sumpin' sumpin' and not family rated. Although this book isn't exactly family rated, but no, not fucking going there.

Open your heart or shine your heart

This is one big fucking UGH. No offense to the fab Neil Diamond, but the heart light is bullshit and we all know it wasn't one of his best. Also in this category, we will file:

Reach your heart to the sky

Shine your heart to the sky

Twist your heart open

Reach your heart forward

No, no, and fuck no. We will do no such thing. Sure, yoga might lighten your load or relieve stress, and it will strengthen your heart the same way other aerobic exercise will. It will in no way illuminate your fucking cardiac muscle. Ain't no E.T. getting down in the fucking yoga studio.

This direction is meant to get you to horizontally lengthen the space beneath your collarbone. I sometimes use *open your shoulders* or *press your sternum forward*. These are both physiologically correct terms and don't induce gagging. I have also instructed clients to give a tiny squeeze between their shoulder blades, but this one can lead to other alignment quirks best avoided. Sit up. Think about your shoulders. Shrug them up to your ears. Yes, I fucking said it. Now roll them back and down. That is opening up your chest. Got it? Good, cuz now I have to go listen to something other than Heartlight so my brain doesn't ooze out of my fucking ears.

Stack your shoulders over your wrist

Fucking ACK! I'll go over this in more detail in the book on asanas, but anyone struggling with carpel tunnel will tell you this is a terrible position. Don't stack your shoulders over anything but your hips while standing. Don't place your wrist at 90 fucking degrees. Trust me.

Awaken Your [insert any body part here]

Okay, at first glance I'm calling bullshit on this one. However, (I'm eye rolling) I have been know to spout, "Say good morning to your hamstring." I'm not 100% certain it qualifies as "Awaken" (said in a breathy, inspirational yoga tone). I do like to say something like, " . . . discover your [insert muscle here] maybe for the first time today or for the first time EVER." I might be splitting hairs, but there you have it.

In this vein, my yoga instructor, the lovely and witty River Cummings, relates the feeling of a stretch in terms of *strength of sensation*. She has a very Zen and calming tone that doesn't make me want to stab anyone because it is truly sincere. It sounds like, "This is a particularly strong stretch." Now, in my lingo that often translates into, "Holy fucking hamsters this is not fun." Po-tay-to, po-tah-to. It's all French fries to me. Mmmmmm, French fries.

Feel Your Anus Blossom

Do I even need to go here? I can't. Just fuck no.

That might cover some of the big culprits of the mumbo jumbo of yoga, but I'm sure you've heard your fair share of stupid shit. Yes, it is stupid. No, you are not alone in thinking that way.

CHAPTER 19

Rockin' Your World: Yoga Schmoga

We can't talk about yoga poses without going back to the idea that physical yoga, the Hatha branch of the eight-limbed practice, wasn't the most important of the whole of yoga. The mindful philosophy is the bedrock of the traditional practice of yoga. If you're confused, go back and fucking review "What The Fuck IS Yoga?" Remember when I said many purists will censure my outlook that a body can practice physical yoga without approaching it from the traditional philosophical angle? I also talked about cultural appropriation in "Namaste, Bitches." I'm stepping out on a fucking limb here (yes, again) and if you're like me it's going to rock your everlovin' world.

There is increasing scholarship and research[1] avowing the origins of the modern physical practice and development of yoga poses were heavily influenced by a Dane[2]. Well, a Dane, a Swede, and a German . . . walk into a bar . . . no, really it isn't a joke. WTF?

---

1   "Those Yoga Poses May Not Be Ancient After All, And Maybe That's OK." *NPR*, NPR, 1 June 2015, www.npr.org/transcripts/411202468.
2   Singleton, Mark. *Yoga Body: the Origins of Modern Posture Practice*. Oxford University Press, 2010.

Wait just a goddamn minute, Julia. You just spent a good portion of this book talking yoga history and philosophy. Thousands of fucking years of yoga. You've linked your practice, albeit unorthodox, to some of the primary intent behind traditional yoga. You've lectured us on using the friggin' Namaste. Respect the yoga tradition, you said. Blah fuckety blah, cultural appropriation, you said. You've sung the praises of Viniyoga to the heavens. What. The. Actual. Fuck?

Fundamentally, all of that is true and I stand by my lectures, but hear me out. I like research. I like to know all of the ins and outs of the things to which I devote energy. Yes, I've read the Christian bible. I've read the Quran. I've studied some of the Torah. You can't know a thing without digging into the vast research and thinking about it all.

The concept that MTPY is relatively young is a theory, and I'm oversimplifying it for the sake of brevity. I've practiced yoga for almost thirty-five years. I've read Patanjali, *Light on Yoga*, and I've studied the Bhagavad Gita. In all of those years, no teacher I've known has offered any more depth to the history of yoga beyond that invented by Tirumalai Krishnamacharya. Seven years ago, my yoga mind was fucking blown, KABOOM, by a yoga scholar named Mark Singleton. He wrote a book called *Yoga Body: The Origins of Modern Posture Practice*. It inspired an even deeper love of yoga in my heart.

Singleton traced the evolution of what we know about modern transnational physical yoga, through the earliest mentions of seated pose and something akin to chair pose (utkatasana) in the Gheranda Samhita (GhS) to Krishnamacharya. A senior researcher in the Department of Languages and Cultures of Southeast Asia at the University of London, Singleton took interest in how yoga became yoga.

The German in this joke, I mean, uh story, was a strongman named Eugen Sandow. Yes, strongmen were a thing. He's famous for his muscle display performances in the late 1800s. He basically invented weightlifting as a physical fitness rather than a fucking sideshow highlight. The Swede in this story, Pehr Ling, developed calisthenics around the same time. You see where this is going? Keep your hands and feet in the fucking cart at all times.

Our next stop is across the North Sea to the land of Beowulf. I give you Niels Bukh, a talented Danish gymnast excluded from the Danish Olympic team in 1908 for being "of thickset and heavy build."[3] (For the record, I could be described this way.) Remember, badasses, body shaming is as old as dirt! He wrote a guide of his own training techniques called *Primary Gymnastics*.[4]

In the late nineteenth century, the idea of physical fitness bloomed as an international movement with the first modern Olympic games. Part of

---

3   Bonde, Hans. *Gymnastics and Politics Niels Bukh and Male Aesthetics*. Museum Tusculanum, 2006.
4   Bukh, Niels. *Grundgymnastik Eller Primitiv Gymnastik*. Hagerups Forlag, 1924.

the reformation of classical education was the belief that physical fitness improved the facility of the mind. The YMCA was founded around this time in England as a response to the cultural upheaval of the British Industrial Revolution. A shift in culture from agricultural to cities and industrial work led to an increase in taverns, gambling houses, and houses of ill-repute. You know, all of the fun shit. YMCA founders believed that given an outlet for physical activity, young men could face the temptations of the industrial world without fucking bending. A fit and healthy temple meant for a clean and spiritually pure mind. A pure mind led to devout faith and devoted public spirit, first-rate subjects for crown and queen. Hmmm, this sounds a lot like traditional yoga.

You still with me after that little road trip? Okay, back to the Village People. Scratch that, back to the British Empire's colonization of the world. Shit, too big. India. We're heading to India.

The Young Men's Christian Association brought its brand of proselytizing and promoting the path to patriotism and the gospel through a robust "body, mind, and spirit" regimen.

Those Scandinavians may have started the modern exercise craze, but the YMCA had the international chops to make it a worldwide thing. Bukh's gymnastic forms traveled well. No weights. No equipment. No special gadgets. Basically, a cheap exercise program that became a boon to an organization preaching physical fitness and religion. Take that, you fucking "yoga is an express ticket to hell" naysayers. Not only that, but Bukh's forms were adopted by the British army and widely introduced in colonial India to the conscripted Indian military as part of their physical training.

Now, imagine a young Tirumalai Krishnamacharya living under an oppressive British regime looking for some inspiration and clinging to his heritage. Okay, it sounds like a bad Brat Pack movie[5] (fuck, I am OLD), but you get the idea.

Like many prophets of old, (Moses, Yahweh, White Buffalo Woman) Krishnamacharya made a pilgrimage into the Himalayan peaks to return with the asanas that now make up the bulk of MTPY. [6]

Mark Singleton compared Bukh's exercises to the Yogasanagalu, the list of Krishnamacharya's yoga poses. The twenty-eight poses (not including variations) are almost identical. Bukh published *Primary Gymnastics* in 1924. Krishnamacharya started demonstrating his asanas in 1926. Obviously, it is more complicated, but if we refuse to acknowledge the complex relationship between conquered and conqueror, we're blindly venerating. I LOVE this kind of shit.

---

5   For those of you under a certain age, the Brat Pack consisted of the baby-faced incarnations of Rob Lowe, Molly Ringwald, Anthony Michael Hall, Emilio Estevez, and Judd Nelson. Google it.

6   There are multiple variations of this story with all of the contradictions and elaborations you might expect when gurus invent themselves.

Interaction between cultures creates a dialogue. Cultural transmission and yoga, baby. I'm talking about the dialogue between the west and the east, loosely designated. Don't let your panties bunch up. There are relatively few (less than a handful), detailed descriptions of the physical yoga poses in the Sutras, and most of those are either seated poses or reclining poses.

If we accept this cultural tryst theory, in my mind, Krishnamacharya pulled the ultimate con on ruling power. He took something intended to conform the native population, added it to the already existing philosophy and asanas, tossed in variations, and linked traditional yoga to a broader physical practice FOREVER. The sublime pot-au-feu he cooked up not only took off in India, but blazed across most of Europe.

As did the YMCA, let's not forget.

Krishnamacharya taught B.K.S. Iyengar, K. Pattabhi Jois, AND my beloved T.K.V. Desikachar. Iyengar and Jois brought yoga to the states and created another firestorm. Now look at MTPY. Who is the fucking conqueror now?

In my humble opinion, the recognition of Bukh's influence on yoga doesn't diminish the practice. It opens the dialogue for a broader discussion on the organic and dynamic entity that yoga is. This tidbit does bring us back to the question of the validity of a purely physical yoga practice. I will go on the fucking record AGAIN and make it clear I am not an expert yoga scholar, but if it looks like a duck, quacks like a duck, and walks like a duck, chances are good it's not a fucking platypus. Without undermining my deference and esteem for the eight-limbed path, I'm gonna say, "Hell yeah." IF you're open minded enough to investigate (and you'll find plenty of traditionalists crying bunk, hocum, and bullshit) it simply means the physical practice of yoga was influenced by BOTH the traditional tenets of the ancient philosophy of yoga and fucking Vikings. Okay, I'm a serious Lagertha fan[7], so influenced by fucking Norsemen happens to work for me.

The complexity of the origins of physical yoga postures leads me to this crazy important question. While working on urdhva mukah svanasana with my class, (upward facing dog) giving my spiel on healthier alignment and positioning (which meant several of them were struggling with the differences between my recommendations and the "traditional" pose as they had been practicing it—some of 'em for years) one of my very dear clients asked, "Why do they teach it that way if there's a better way to perform it?"

The simple stupid answer is *because*.

Because Krishnamacharya, by all accounts was an alignment Nazi who used sticks to beat his students into the "correct" position. His yoga was strict and idealized without taking into account a student's individual body. *Because* his students, Iyengar and Jois had their own idealized and fairly

---

7 This is a reference to the television series, *Vikings* and the very real 12th century shield-maiden from what is now known as Norway.

rigid concepts when they brought yoga to the west. *Because*, frankly, there is such an aura of sacrosanct bullshit surrounding yoga and its practice that a lot of people don't question what an instructor tells them to do. Even if it hurts them to do it. These exercises (if we're taking Neils Bukh into account, and I am) were designed for gymnasts—serious fucking gymnasts—who generally have a completely different physiology than mere mortals. I also have several former gymnast clients who have beaten the shit out of their bodies to transcend mere mortalhood. Some of these poses as traditionally taught, aren't good for the body.

Even the *Gheranda Samhita* states only 32 were suited for human beings. A lot of yoga programs don't require more than basic anatomy and that doesn't guarantee an understanding of healthy alignment or kinesiology (the study of the mechanics of body movements). The commercialization, rebranding, and repackaging of yoga creates all kinds of wibbly wobbly quackery. Many yoga programs have developed the focus on "pushing yourself" and "cowboy up" practices. Honestly, it's because the majority of western yoga practitioners just don't have the interest or patience for what they consider a non-workout. Americans in particular, always seem to be looking for the stronger, faster, harder exercise fad.

I'm not going to trash any one thing, but client after client come to me injured or recovering from some crazy ass workout that tore them up.

Shoulder injuries, knee injuries, hip injuries, back injuries. We are obsessed with the idea that exercise must torment in order to be effective. To be fair, I teach cycle. It is friggin' excruciating. Every single time; and I teach it three, sometimes four, times a week. If you have good form, if you refrain from doing something on the stationary bike you wouldn't do on a bicycle, if you're fucking MINDFUL, it's great. Not great while you're doing it, understand. Great after about an hour, a hot shower, and maybe a double espresso.

What's the fucking point of resisting the consecrated idea that yoga is an inviolable tradition? Well first, I would like to repeat that approaching yoga with humility is a good place to start. Opening up to the possibility that yoga isn't hallowed and saintly is the epitome of humble. Learn a bit about its traditional philosophical history so you can respect its origins and its rich culture. They are worthy of it. Then, figure out what works for you. If following the path to Bhakti yoga floats your boat, bon voyage. If the eight-limbed path looks like the route for you, go ohm. Heh, heh. If you can find a mindful physical practice that serves you with the highest and conscientious of intentions, fucking rock it.

The point in introducing the Vikings into the discussion is threefold. One, it's a valid theory with evidence to support it. Two, I like it. I like it because it's complex and chewy. It allows wiggle room and support for the physical practice. And three (this is a big one) it gives me license to say, "Stop being so fucking snooty about your goddamn yoga."

I, myself, am wary of torches and pitchforks any time the subject arises in hippy dippy yogi company. You think yoga people are all Zen and shit, but like any zealot they can go fucking rabid. Don't kid yourself.

Like I really needed an excuse to say that, but I'll take any validation I can get. There is no "real" yoga outside of the philosophical practice of Ashtanga, the eight-limbed path. That doesn't mean all yoga is good yoga. Cuz it's not. I'm embracing Satya (truthfulness) and looking to encourage Aparigraha, (non-greed or non-possessiveness in others). It's a work in progress.

CHAPTER 20

Slow Your Roll, Bitches

We've all heard it and sure, most of you ignore it, but a good warm-up before a workout is all kinds of good for your body. Yoga isn't the exception. In fact, I'd argue (and I will), that it's hella more important to warm-up to a yoga pose than any other workout. I've already scolded you (in many previous chapters) on not stretching after a hardcore routine. Warming up dilates your blood vessels and increases your oxygen delivery system. Remember, "I AM Breathing, Bitch?" As you warm up, you start revving up your respiratory system, thus, gearing up to full activation of said respiratory system and adding more oxygen to that delivery system. You raise your body temperature as you ease muscles into working mode. You work the kinks and creaks out of the body so you can amp up your heart rate. Basically, you are getting the bod ready to be more efficient and less prone to injury.

Duh.

Someone said, "Try yoga it will change your life." They fail to mention the first few classes will suck eggs. In case you missed it the first few times, yoga is the long con. If you are reading this book, it's likely you fucking hate yoga. And one of the biggest reasons is that you are not flexible. If I haven't convinced you yet, you don't walk into any yoga class and ace shit. I live in an area where three growing cities are slowly merging into one metropolitan area. We have two universities and two community colleges. I estimate we have almost sixty yoga studios in an area with approximately 387,000 people. Consider my town of only 25,000 people; we've got two yoga studios, a Pilates studio, a recreation center—and count 'em—five gyms. I'm pretty sure every one of those places offers a yoga class of some kind.

I am the only teacher within the tri-city area population of 387,000 people who offers a beginning yoga class. I did look that up. Sure, several studios offer gentle yoga, but all of those studios claim every one of their classes are suitable for beginners. Bullshit. Imma say it again, bullshit.

I go to yoga classes. I see how they are managed. Only three or four teachers in the last fifteen years I've lived in the area were cognizant of and welcoming to beginners. All of them a part of the Viniyoga team, these people taught my certification program. Without fail, every other yoga class I've attended targeted the experienced yogi without modification or consideration of the diverse attendees.

I usually prefer to go incognito. I don't tell those instructors that I am also a yoga instructor. I got a story. Would you like to hear it? It goes like this:

Once upon a time, I belonged to a chi chi health club. Yes, they had white fluffy towels and a pool. I had been teaching yoga in my area about ten years. I don't know if you can imagine, but I'm not really a wallflower. I was dipping into some of the yoga classes at the club to shift up my practice. I had been a couple of times to a particular class with an instructor also named Julia. Go figure. Now, I didn't love how fast she was guiding the flow and I had slowed down a bit to fit my mojo. (This clearly irritated her. Remember what I said about control freaks?), but I was paying for the fancy club and I told you, I like to go to as many classes to fit my $5 per class price point. To be fair, I didn't hate her flows. She just had a lead foot.

On this day, four of my regular yoga clients walked into the room. I guess they had some special offer, you know, a free week of classes to sweeten the idea of joining. I've already mentioned Randy but I'll call out to his wife, Carla whom I adore. They were two of the four. They see me and start a clamor. Hugs all around. Isn't this a coincidence? It didn't go unnoticed by the other Julia. She walks over to see what the hell is the deal and my clients explain.

"So YOU'RE the Julia I keep hearing about?" She says. "People keep asking me if I'm The Julia and I guess you are who they are talking about."

It's all amusing and lighthearted until she starts class . . . and proceeds to kick everyone's ass. I'm telling you, I had been to her class three or four times, but the minute she discovered I'm THAT Julia, she ratcheted her flow up. Remember yoga teacher ego? Yeah, it may have been subconscious, but she was proving to me how serious her yoga kung fu was. I watched the rest of class struggle through the hour. She brutalized her clients to prove something to herself and possibly to me.

She isn't the only yogini to do it.

That Screaming Mimi yoga Nazi? The drill sergeant? The minute she discovered I taught yoga, same exact thing. She ignored the well-being of her clients to show me her superior yoga skills. In both instances, I saw people injuring themselves to keep up.

I am wary of any yoga class labeled with "all levels are welcome." I'm a former school teacher. I'm trained to teach to the lowest twenty-five percent of the room. I have a Masters Degree in Education with the skills to teach to a variety of students. I apply this principle to my beginning yoga class. I am here to serve my clients with the highest purpose of doing no harm. That is sadly not the case in many yoga classes.

I've said it before and I'll keep saying it: a fitness instructor can injure you. Yoga teachers are no exception, and in some cases, they are worse.

Ten percent of folks who try yoga experience injuries. Another twenty-one percent will aggravate existing pain. Sure, yoga will change your life and sometimes NOT for the better. *Well shit, Julia. Tell me again why I should do yoga? You're not really selling me here.* It's my job to create a series of poses that will serve you for the better. I'm not here to blow smoke up your skirt.

I'm blurring the lines between yoga Nazis and yoga bitches here; bear with me. Imagine that shitty yoga class you've attended. Picture that super svelte, very young yoga ingénue. Yeah, I kinda hate her too. With love. I hate with love! She's throwing her body into the extreme version of every pose to prove to the instructor and to everyone around her, how amazing her yoga is. It's a chain reaction. She has been to many yoga classes, all teaching the same yoga bullshit and now she's bumped into me, this crazy, tattooed bitch telling her almost everything she knows is wrong. Ego. Yes, I struggle with ego, if you hadn't noticed.

It happens on the reg. Once they see me or hear my spiel, the light dies in their eyes a little. Not only are my alignment cues wonky, I'm not impressed by their contortions. By nature, young bodies are more flexible, in fact, they tend to be hyper flexible, which isn't a good thing. I refer you back to "My Dog Doesn't Do Downward" here. As we grow older, shit starts to dry out and stiffen up—not in a good way.

I don't care if you can launch your body into the strongest expression of eka pada ustrasana (*ey-kuh pah-duh oosh-trahs-anna*) (single leg camel pose) in a blink.

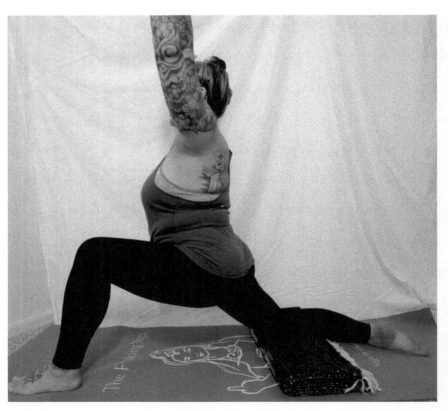

Sequencing is as important as healthy alignment. That's where so many yoga classes jump the fucking shark and where Viniyoga has your back. Literally. The focus on spinal health and joint movement means warming the body up to stronger poses and bringing the energy back. Think about a six-on-the-floor Porsche 911. Some of you will have to look that up, I'll wait. Okay, okay, for you young 'uns, it harkens back to dinosaur days when automobiles had manual transmissions rather than automatic ones.

You accelerated and increased the RPMs gradually. Only then, could you take your foot off of the gas and press the clutch to shift into a higher gear. You moved from first gear to second to third as the vehicle accelerated. Your body is exactly like that Porsche 911, yeah it is. Own it, bitches. Sure, those of you in newer models might be able to go from zero to sixty in two-point-nine seconds, but you still have to shift through the gears. If you slam into fourth gear from first, you are going to stall out the engine. The reverse is also true. If you drop from fifth to first without going through the motions, you are going to drop your tranny[1].

All of my flows build the heat and move the body in preparation for that power surge.

Driving a stick shift also includes skillful application of the clutch so you can move through neutral without grinding the gears. Remember, we're fucking Porsches. We don't want any costly repairs. In yoga, neutral is a forward fold. As we move from asana to asana, we have to offer the body a neutral position to shift our spinal movement. In *Yoga for Wellness*, Gary Kraftsow reminds us, "From a biomechanics perspective, according to

---

1   For those of you who cringed, this is a reference to your transmission. One of my childhood friends did this exact thing in his bright, metallic blue Z28. It ain't pretty.

Viniyoga tradition, the primary intention of forward folding is to stretch the structure of the lumbo-sacral spine."

That's your low back, homies. We all experience low back pain. Some of us more than others. A lot of yoga flows can be designed with specific goals. Whether it's a forward folding practice or a lateral extension practice or a twisting practice, in order to accommodate safe shifting from pose to pose, you have to hit that neutral position. No stripping the gears in my yoga class.

The other thing to take into consideration is the heat. The more we warm up parts of our bodies, the more we notice tension in other areas. In Morning Energy Yoga this particular morning, I introduced some shoulder and Latissimus Dorsi action into our flow. I added a little garudasana (*gahr-oo-dahs-uh-nuh*) arm (eagle pose) after we warmed up with some cactus arm and large arm circles.

One round of eagle arm, and I could add the first round of the arm bind in standing parsvottanasana (*parsh-voh-than-ahs-anna*) (pyramid pose) as the counter stretch to those round shoulders.

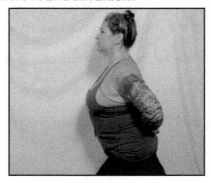

After we repeated that flow a couple of times, I added an ardha puras utkatasana (*are-duh purr-ahs oot-kah-tahs-anna* - forward folding chair pose) and the low back release was crazy! We had warmed up our shoulder girdles. We had lengthened and loosened our Latissimus Dorsi. Creating length and warming up those other parts allowed us to get a little longer in our lumbar structure. That's the beauty of sequencing. As my father used to say, "Patience, jackass." Sure, it's irritating as hell for some folks and in this age of instantaneous results, going the low and slow route might not appeal. Look, I'm the first one to experience first-world problem rage when my Wi-Fi is dinking along. But yoga ain't your Wi-Fi connection.

That's why yoga, done correctly and with healthy intent, is the long con.

I think we can all agree everything is better with a little lubrication. That includes your joint and muscle movement.

Moving through a sequence in repetition also adds to the ooey gooey of the mind. We're back to talking the whole intent of yoga. This moving meditation jam gives you room to work the noise out of your mind while lubing up the body. It's a twofer! This is also where I'm still struggling with the "you can do an effective flow in twenty minutes" theory.

I'm not saying never. That's sure to bite me in the ass.

Look, I'm happy to get my sunshine, vitamin D mojo on in twenty minutes. Ten minutes each side, baby. I have been known to grab a quick twenty-minute snooze. I can toss the shit I need for a smoothie in the blender in less than twenty minutes. I certainly don't want to spend more than twenty minutes paying bills. And damn, I'm a fan of the don't clean shit for longer than twenty minutes even if it means some of the dust bunnies escape.

Let's face it, anything really worth the time is worth spending more than twenty minutes. Making a great meal. Taking the pups for a walk. Hanging out with friends. Drinking a bottle of wine. Sex only takes longer than twenty minutes in the movies.

I have my priorities.

Brahmacharya, bitches; it's the channeling and managing the energy within, toward greater personal connection. I'm working on it. Or *Tapas* . . . no, not the snack, though I dig me some of those as well! I'm talking one of the five Niyamas. *Tapas* means to cultivate our inner sense of discipline and wisdom. Take your pick, but either way, slow your roll.

CHAPTER 21

You Want Me to Put My Foot Where?

The names of the poses in MTPY come from Indian mythology, animals, and are sometimes pulled out of a yoga teacher's ass. In Vinyoga, poses are categorized as forward bending, backward bending (not always what you think), twisting, lateral extension, core extensions, inversions, and balances. You'll find standing poses, seated poses, supine poses, and prone poses. This is where twenty-eight poses turns into something like three hundred. And it has to be said; one pose can go by several different names. So that's easy, right? Bullshit.

You'll need a couple of directional references to wrap your head around before we step onto the mat. Think of one end of your mat as true north. I say *true* because any of you out there with navigational experience knows there's True and Magnetic. I'm trying to be precise here, so get a fucking grip. We'll start with longitude. Okay, imagine you're standing face outward (anterior), about ten inches from the true north end of your mat.

We generally step from this standing position to other poses. When we talk about the front and back of the mat, we can move in two directions, forward and back. You have a long stance (an elongated distance between your feet front to back) or a short stance, (a compressed distance between your feet front to back. Duh). Long stance. Short stance. The verbal cue sounds like this: "Lengthen your stance, or if you're feeling off balance, shorten your stance."

In Transverse Plane, we're talking latitude. That refers to the width of your stance. You can have a wide stance (feet apart laterally) or a narrow stance (feet together). Wide stance. Narrow stance. In a yoga studio with floorboards, I usually say, "Standing on train tracks" to get folks to widen their stance. I teach my clients to place their feet "a little wider than fist width." It's technically neutral stance, in terms of Pilates.

Four directions, okay? Front to back and side-to-side. Yes, you will have to remember those when we're upside down. Yes, we sometimes stand and hang upside down at the same time. Don't panic.

Expression is another term I use you might remember from the "Mumbo Jumbo" chapter. I like this word because it considers the difference in how each person might exist IN a pose. I like to demonstrate modifications to first-time clients to remove the pressure of striving for something that won't serve their body. After that I may say, "The full expression of this pose looks like . . ." Or maybe, "A stronger expression would be . . ." This is more common in my beginning class because I like clients to know where they are headed. I also use it when approaching challenging poses. Expression is about flavoring your yoga with individual alignment and placement. No such thing as fucking perfect pose!

A lot of yoga is taught with a narrow stance or feet aligned one behind the other. My alignment instruction is a direct departure from this particular foot placement. When standing in neutral position, remember to have your feet a little wider than fist-width. You are not in control if you are out of balance. If your feet are pressed together or aligned like you're standing on a balance beam, you are NOT in a balanced stance. It's like a sobriety test. Some folks can barely pull that heel-to-toe shit off sober, let alone after a drink or two. If I can push you over, you're out of fucking balance. I get a lot of questions about this foot placement thing from clients with yoga experience. WHY, they ask. Why do we learn it this way in the first place? Because. While "because" is a good enough for some English grammar rules (it's a wonky language), it's not good enough for your yoga placement. I instruct clients to place their feet in alignment with their hips. Remember though, not the widest point of the iliac crests, but the lower, anterior iliac spines. This is one aspect of neutral posture.

It's a general rule and we are not the same. Not one of us. Maybe you have knee issues. I have a couple of clients who are bowlegged. I have one who is knock-kneed. Your foot placement might need adjustments. In addition to *feet on railroad tracks*, I cue parallel placement of the feet. Some folks naturally or habitually turn out their feet. This is often more to do with tight hamstrings and glutes. Some folks stand with their toes turned in a bit, a likely result from tight adductors or hip flexors. My point is, standing in a truly neutral position will feel wonky as fuck for a while. I'll say it again. It took a long time for us to get into our current physical condition and it will take a while to make changes.

The second biggest issue for yoga folks in my classes is the shoulders. Okay, to be fair, everyone has problems with this shoulder business. I'm going to tell you a little secret. You ready? Your shoulders can move independently of your arms, your ribs, your hips, your spine, AND your neck. Isn't that cool? I don't make this shit up. Try it out. Give 'em a little shrug. Move them forward. Pull them back. They also move independently of each other. No fucking lie. The body is an amazing piece of machinery.

Let's play a game. Wherever you are, think about your posture. (Everyone immediately sat up straight, or rather, what you all think is straight.) Sit someplace you can put your feet all of the way on the ground. Move a bit to the edge if you must. Line your knees up with the center of your hips (those iliac spines) or measure your fist between your knees. Don't squeeze your knees, let them rest outside of your fist. Add a little less than an inch on each side of your fist. Lift and spread your toes. Now, sit up as tall as you can. To open the space up under your collarbone, rotate your shoulders away from the center of your chest. Give a little squeeze between your shoulder blades and engage your abdominal muscles. Relax your fucking shoulders. Tuck your chin just a smidge. Are you working? Damn straight you are. This is neutral alignment. Good posture.

There's a reason for the expression, "looking down your nose at someone." Those considered "higher stature" used to take lessons in polite behavior. (I obviously skipped those lessons.) That included good posture. Yes, your mother was right. Sit up straight! We're a modern society of slouchers. We could call it the good selfie rule. I always thought if I lifted my chin I looked thinner. False! The only thing folks can see is a primo view of my fucking nostrils. Tuck your chin to ninety degrees. Think about pressing your head and neck backward to touch the collar of a shirt. Okay, an imaginary shirt because I don't have many shirts with collars.

Relax a minute. Go ahead and slouch.

Now, move back into that neutral posture. Start with your legs and hips. Think about your feet. Rotate your shoulders back and engage your abdominals. Get a little taller. Think about doing all of that while on a yoga mat. It's a lot. I know. That's why yoga ain't for sissies.

Let's go back to your shoulders. It's not just that people don't really understand how their shoulders move, it's the feeling that lifting their shoulders makes them feel like they've lengthened their spine. Shoulders are also the first place we trap stress. They creep up toward our ears. Relax your shoulders. Heh heh, see? Seasoned yoga people struggle with their shoulders in my class for different reasons. Mostly to do with traditional expressions of postures, but we'll get into that in book two.

I know I keep saying it, but it's important. Physical yoga is about renewing a relationship with your body. And the bloody shame is many yoga teachers aren't facilitating that intimacy.

So, you ready to step on the fucking mat?

CHAPTER 22

Balancing the Zing with the Zen

The foundation of my yoga practice is Viniyoga. I've gushed about TKV Desikachar and Gary Kraftsow, not sorry if you're tired of hearing it. Build a bridge, bitches. Viniyoga is about recovery, wellness, and adaptation. If you take anything away from this book, beside my passion for profanity (something proven by scientific study to be linked with higher fucking intelligence, btw. Go science!) and booze (shhhhhh), let it be this: I don't have to do everything a fitness instructor tells me to do, especially if it causes me fucking pain.

There's a difference between pain and discomfort. Remember that upward facing dog class? Where my "I wish she was my mother" Carla asked me the *why* question? There was a lot of push back on my instruction. There is always push back because my direction is not what most people find familiar. The most common reason given is, "It doesn't feel right." *Hold up Julia, didn't you just say we don't have to do everything a fitness instructor tells us to do?* Yes, I did.

In this case, it's a matter of change versus habit. A lot of yoga practitioners rely on muscle memory and habit to "hang out" in their poses. If you are not finding a way to grow stronger in a pose, what purpose does it serve? One of my younger clients waited after this up-dog session to ask me about lotus pose.

"I was wondering what you recommend for approaching lotus pose more successfully?"

"Um, back away slowly without making any sudden movements and when you're clear, run like you fucking stole it." I said.

Okay, I was only sort of joking. If you can do lotus pose, great, more power to you. Frankly, there are a shit ton of poses I don't even consider doing. I'm 50-plus years old. In this case, I challenged my young client by asking, "How is that pose serving you? Does it improve anything for you?"

She was flummoxed. There was no answer. Well, you know there is one. Fucking Ego.

I ain't sitting in lotus pose. Lotus pose is that sitting pretzel pose most people associate with yoga; legs crossed with each foot tucked on top of each thigh and your hands forming the gyan mudra (the okay symbol turned palm up on the knees). I have a weak knee, humongous calves, tight hips, and a powerful appreciation for the feeling in my feet. All of these things are better served by other seated poses. I like to take seated meditation in a modified version of sukhasana (*soo-kaah-sun-ah*), also known as easy or pleasant pose. Think of crisscross applesauce without stacking your legs on top of your feet. I can balance my weight on my sit bones (lower ischial tuberosities, for those who are technically minded), relax my legs completely, lengthen my spine, and my hips don't bitch. I'm supposed to be removing the focus on the body, not wrestling it into fucking submission.

This gorgeous young woman could easily get into half lotus, (one foot tucked on top of a thigh) but she wasn't evenly balanced. Her left hip was tight, keeping her knee higher and causing more tension in her hip. She listed to one side as a result. Her posture slumped. I don't know many average practitioners who can lengthen their spine in lotus or even half-lotus. Are there folks out there sitting like gods and goddesses in lotus pose? Fuck yeah. Absolutely. This earth mama ain't one of them. In my yoga world, the benefit of the pose must outweigh any other factor INCLUDING ego. Seriously, I don't care what fucking hippy dippy, chakra bullshit you offer me in the way of justification; there is zero physical benefit to being able to lift your leg to parallel your ear. Except to be a douchebag showoff. I am embracing Satya, the act of truthfulness and encouraging Aparigraha, letting go of want or the embracing the act of non-grasping here.

Another pose I don't do is ustrasana (a form of camel pose). This version requires standing on your knees in a backbend. I have had at least twenty different yoga instructors tell me they have the perfect approach for me to get into this pose. And fifteen of those times, I've let them con me into believing it. After those attempts, I've spent two or three weeks with painful back issues. Ustrasana doesn't serve me, and I see absolutely zero benefit in going there. Now, can other people achieve camel pose without any issues? You betcha and they're welcome to it.

Fear definitely keeps me from some poses, but some poses are non-starters. Dhyana is being aware without focus, the act of letting go. I'm working on it.

With my background of injury and my weird ass synchronicity with the philosophy of Viniyoga, I approach poses in a way that challenges without ravaging a body. Each pose is different for a lot of average yoga goers.

Second verse same as the first; spinal health is the crux of the Viniyoga brand (that and sequencing), but we're talking spine. You can revisit "Baby Got Back" for the nitty gritty. My approach to poses always takes into account the spine and the core. Pilates, dontcha fucking know. I will harp and harp and harp on healthy alignment, stability and balance, and being in control till doomsday. I'm hoping that is much later than sooner. I think I've been pretty clear about all of the ways a yoga teacher can fuck up your practice, even with the best of intentions. Need I mention the road to hell?

If you have a long-standing yoga practice and give my corrections a shot, you're going to feel wonky as fuck. That's the difference between habit and awareness. Here's a hypothetical: have you ever driven home from work without even realizing how you arrived? That's fucking habit; same goes for yoga. Habit is mindless. It's empty. It's easy. I'm going back to the traditional tenets of yoga here. Dharana and dhyana are the opposite of habit. This is where I believe the physical practice of yoga can move you into all of the groovy aspects of the philosophical intentions. Dharana is the immovable focus of attention. We can link breath to body and yoke[1] our concentration to that connection.

Dhyana is the shifting of concentration to contemplation. We can be ardently aware of our practice without any effort. This is where our movement blurs into meditation. Mindfulness and stillness. If we want to jump into the deep end of the fucking pool, we can call it samadhi; the body and senses at rest while the mind and reason are alert in meditative consciousness. This is what traditional practitioners argue as the primary goal of yoga.

It's the fucking bomb.

Another bullshit thing earning me a spot on the yoga blacklist is my informed opinion that many yoga poses serve no purpose. Sure, they boost

---

1   My bad. I have completely forgotten an important definition. The word yoga comes from the Sanskrit word *yuj* which means to yoke or to bind. This is often interpreted to mean union. Union of body, breath, and movement. Union to the divine. Union of the internal with the external. Union of the Yamas. Take your pick.

your ego, but I'm talking actual physical benefit. I'm not against doing things that inspire your inner badass. (I have one tattoo that starts at the base of my neck and flows down to my ankles. I would carry a broadsword but the hubby isn't sure that would fly. Now that would inspire my inner badass. He did buy me throwing knives. No worries, I'll be firing up my warrior ninja skills soon.)

In yoga, it would be refreshing not to see a photo of some yogi performing urdhva janu sirsasana (*oord-vah jah-new shear-shahs-anna*) (upward head to knee pose) as an iconic image of yoga. This is pure ego unless you have a life goal of joining Cirque de Soleil. Okay, they're badasses but I'm talking about the rest of us. There are many benefits to doing this pose as basic head to knee without your leg up by your ear. Many of the bound versions of poses are also ego-fests. Not only do they fail to provide physical benefit, many of those poses fuck up your alignment (often you have to twist and wrench to get into these binds) and that can cause injuries.

Let me add to this list: many of the arm balances, fish pose, full locust pose, etcetera. It should be noted, a lot of these poses have modifications so you can do them with benefits. In the end, yoga must serve you. You have to feel better about yourself and the challenge of simply stepping onto the mat without being discouraged. We all have room to improve but look away from the yoga magazine that shall not be named.

The reality is very few of us are in any kind of shape to being doing some of these ridiculous poses and there are even fewer instructors with enough physiology or biology training to understand the consequences of encouraging such poses. Yoga is amazing. It's the fucking bomb. Under the best circumstances it is challenging.

This is yoga for the rest of us.

BIBLIOGRAPHY

Andrew, Elise. "Why You Can Blame Evolution For Your Back Ache." IFLScience, IFLScience, 11 Mar. 2019, www.iflscience.com/health-and-med-icine/evolution-blame-lower-back-pain/.

A.s.ayyavu. "In Indian Culture Why Do We Do Namaste or Greet Each Other?" In Indian Culture Why Do We Do Namaste or Greet Each Other?, 19 Mar. 2014, legacyofwisdom.blogspot.com/2014/03/in-indian-culture-why-do-we-do-namaste.html.

Bard, W. "Five Factors That Affect Your Flexibility." Wellness Focus, 27 Nov. 2017, svmassagetherapy.com/blog/2015/06/16/five-factors-affect-flexibili-ty/.

"Benefits of Yoga." American Osteopathic Association, www.osteopathic.org/osteopathic-health/about-your-health/health-conditions-library/gener-al-health/Pages/yoga.aspx.

Bharati, Swami Jnaneshvara. "Modern Yoga versus Traditional Yoga." Yoga Meditation, www.swamij.com/traditional-yoga.htm. Accessed 12 Mar. 2017

Bharati, Swami Jananeshvara. "Yoga and Institutional Religion - Insight for Yoga Meditation." Yoga Meditation, www.swamij.com/yoga-institutional-religion.htm. Accessed 7 Feb. 2017.

Black, Lindsey I, et al. "Use of Yoga, Meditation, and Chiropractors Among U.S. Children Aged 4-17 Years." NCHS Data Brief, U.S. National Library of Medicine, Nov. 2018, www.ncbi.nlm.nih.gov/pubmed/30475687.

"Booze Myths Uncovered, No.4: Sweating out a Hangover." JOE.ie, JOE, 1 June 2013, www.joe.ie/uncategorized/booze-myths-uncovered-no4-sweating-out-a-hangover/37105.

Bouchez, Colette. "Yoga for Weight Loss?" WebMD, WebMD, 2006, www.webmd.com/fitness-exercise/features/yoga-for-weight-loss#1.

Bradford, Alina. "Lungs: Facts, Function and Diseases." LiveScience, Purch, 1 Feb. 2018, www.livescience.com/52250-lung.html.

Burgin, Timothy. "Bhakti Yoga: the Yoga of Devotion • Yoga Basics." Yoga Basics, 1 Apr. 2020, www.yogabasics.com/learn/bhakti-yoga-the-yoga-of-devotion/.

Carrico, Mara. "Get to Know the Eight Limbs of Yoga." Yoga Journal, 28 Aug. 2007, www.yogajournal.com/article/beginners/the-eight-limbs/.

Coleman, Erin. "Calories Burned for Yoga: Is It Enough for Weight Loss? / Fitness / Cardio." / Fitness / Cardio, www.fitday.com/fitness-articles/fitness/cardio/calories-burned-for-yoga-is-it-enough-for-weight-loss.html.

Costello, Nikki. "The Subtle Struggle of Savasana." Yoga Journal, 15 Nov. 2013, www.yogajournal.com/article/beginners/corpse-pose/.

Cramer, Holger, et al. "A Systematic Review of Yoga for Major Depressive Disorder."

Journal of Affective Disorders, U.S. National Library of Medicine, 15 Apr. 2017, www.ncbi.nlm.nih.gov/pubmed/28192737.

Cummins, Claudia. "Six Different Views on Breathing in Yoga." Yoga Journal, 28 Aug. 2007, www.yogajournal.com/article/practice-section/prescriptions-for-pranayama/.

Desikachar, T. K. V. The Heart of Yoga: Developing a Personal Practice. Inner Traditions International, 1999.

Editors, YJ. "Corpse Pose." Yoga Journal, 28 Aug. 2007, www.yogajournal.com/pose/corpse-pose/.

Friedrich, Guts Muths Johann Christoph, and Schröder Willi. Gymnastik für Die Jugend: Enthaltend Eine Praktische Anweisung Zu Leibesübungen: Ein Beytrag Zurnöthigsten Verbesserung Der körperlichen Erziehung. Hain, Verlag, 1999.

Garrouste, Christelle. 100 Years of Educational Reforms in Europe: a Contextual Database . European Union, 2010, pp. 1–112, https://publications.jrc.ec.europa.eu/repository/bitstream/JRC57357/reqno_jrc57357.pdf.

Gerber, Toni, and Susan Ince. "Do You Need Back Surgery?" Good Housekeeping, 9 Apr. 2017.

Grazioplene, Rachael. "This Is Your Brain on Yoga." Psychology Today, Sussex Publishers, Sept. 2012, www.psychologytoday.com/us/blog/quilted-science/201209/is-your-brain-yoga.

Grinspoon, Peter. "Medical Marijuana." Harvard Health Blog, 9 Jan. 2018, www.health.harvard.edu/blog/medical-marijuana-2018011513085.

Guimaraes, Thais. "Top 10 Yoga Cue Translations: Flutter My What?" YogaDork, 16 Nov. 2011, yogadork.com/2011/11/15/top-10-yoga-cue-translations-flutter-my-what/.

Harvard Health Publishing. "Calories Burned in 30 Minutes for People of Three Different Weights." Harvard Health, Aug. 2018, www.health.harvard.edu/newsweek/Calories-burned-in-30-minutes-of-leisure-and-routine-activities.htm.

Harvard Health Publishing. "Relaxation Techniques: Breath Control Helps Quell Errant Stress Response." Harvard Health, 2016, www.health.harvard.edu/mind-and-mood/relaxation-techniques-breath-control-helps-quell-errant-stress-response.

Heinz, Erica. "Staying Grounded: Not Just Another Yoga Cliche." The Huffington Post, TheHuffingtonPost.com, 17 Nov. 2011, www.huffingtonpost.com/erica-heinz/yoga-poses-staying-ground_b_538779.html.

Iyengar, B. K. S., and Patañjali. Light on the Yoga Sūtras of Patañjali. Harper Collins, 2005.

Konie, Robin. "Ten Beautiful Lessons Learned from Savasana." Thank Your Body, 12 Sept. 2019, www.thankyourbody.com/lessons-from-savasana/.

Kraft, Amy. "Reality Check: Does Yoga Release Toxins from the Body?" CBS News, CBS Interactive, 15 Apr. 2016, www.cbsnews.com/news/reality-check-yoga-does-not-release-toxins-from-the-body/.

Lewis, Dennis. "Some Facts About Deep Breathing." Dennis Lewis, 13 July 2015, www.dennislewis.org/articles-other-writings/articles-essays/some-facts-about-deep-breathing/.

Lovely, Lori. "The Line between Cultural Appropriation and Cultural Appreciation." NUVO, 25 Oct. 2019, www.nuvo.net/voices/guestvoices/the-line-between-cultural-appropriation-and-cultural-appreciation/article_c0503f24-f712-11e9-ad9e-93d5c3a43bea.html.

Marksberry, Kellie. "Take a Deep Breath." The American Institute of Stress, 4 Jan. 2017, www.stress.org/take-a-deep-breath/.

Matt Gill. "The Benefits of Yoga for Feet." Matt Gill, Matt Gill, 16 Feb. 2018, mattgillyoga.co.uk/blog/2018/2/16/the-benefits-of-yoga-for-feet.

McCall, Timothy, M.d. "38 Health Benefits of Yoga." Yoga Journal, 28 Aug. 2007, www.yogajournal.com/lifestyle/count-yoga-38-ways-yoga-keeps-fit.

Metcalf, Eric Acosta, et al. "Foot Health - Don't Tiptoe Around Its Importance: Everyday Health." EverydayHealth.com, 13 Apr. 2009, www.everydayhealth.com/foot-health/foot-health-basics.aspx.

Miller, Richard. "10 Steps of Yoga Nidra." Yoga Journal, 27 Jan. 2013, www.yogajournal.com/article/practice-section/10-steps-of-yoga-nidra/.

Mohan, A. G., and Ganesh Mohan. Krishnamacharya: His Life and Teachings. Shambhala, 2010.

Muddagouni, Kamna. "Why White People Need to Stop Saying 'Namaste'." The Sydney Morning Herald, The Sydney Morning Herald, 1 Apr. 2016, www.smh.com.au/lifestyle/news-and-views/social/why-white-people-need-tostop-saying-namaste-20160401-gnw2xx.html.

"Namaste: It's Philosophy and Significance in Indian Culture." ReligionFacts, 29 Oct. 2016, www.religionfacts.com/namaste.

"Noninvasive Nonpharmacological Treatment for Chronic Pain: A Systematic Review." Effective Health Care Program, 11 June 2018, effectivehealthcare. ahrq.gov/topics/nonpharma-treatment-pain/research-2018.

Osborn, Lisa Mae. "A Word About Namaste." The Bhakti Yoga Movement Center, The Bhakti Yoga Movement Center, 28 May 2019, thebhaktiyogam-ovementcenter.com/bhaktimusings/a-word-about-namaste.

PATANJALI. YOGA SUTRAS OF PATANJALI. DIGIREADS COM, 2017.

Payne Ph. D, Larry. "The Father of Modern Yoga." The Huffington Post, TheHuffingtonPost.com, 7 Dec. 2017, www.huffingtonpost.com/larry-payne-phd/yoga-history_b_3009822.html.

"Pranayama Exercises & Poses." Yoga Journal, 3 Apr. 2017, www.yogajournal.com/category/poses/types/pranayama/.

"Pranayama: The Beginner's Guide to Yoga Breathing Exercises." Art of Living (United States), www.artofliving.org/us-en/yoga/breathing-tech-niques/yoga-and-pranayama.

Rodriguez-Rojas, Ivanna C. "Fetishization for Dummies: Columbia Edition." Columbia Daily Spectator, 1 2018, www.columbiaspectator.com/opinion/2018/11/01/fetishization-for-dummies-columbia-edition/.

Ruiz, Fernando Pagés. "Krishnamacharya's Legacy: Modern Yoga's Inventor." Yoga Journal, 28 Aug. 2007, www.yogajournal.com/article/philosophy/krishnamacharya-s-legacy/.

Sargeant, Winthrop, and Christopher Key Chapple. The Bhagavad Gītā. State University of New York Press, 1994.

Seppälä, Emma. "Benefits of Breathing: The Scientific Benefits of Breathing INFOGRAPHIC." Emma Seppälä, Ph.D., 11 Aug. 2017, www.emmaseppala.com/benefits-breathing-scientific-benefits-breathing-infographic/.

Singh, Roopa Bala. "We Are Not Exotic, We Are Exhausted: South Asian Diasporic Youth Speak." South Asian American Perspectives on Yoga in America (SAAPYA), 19 Nov. 2014, saapya.wordpress.com/2014/11/19/we-are-not-exoticwe-are-exhausted-south-asian-diasporic-youth-speak/.

Singleton, Mark. Yoga Body: the Origins of Modern Posture Practice. Oxford University Press, 2010.

Shapiro, Nina L. "Take a Deep Breath." 2012, doi:10.1142/9789814343794.

Slavin, Nicole. "Demystifying Detox: Can Yoga Really Cleanse the Liver?" The Guardian, Guardian News and Media, 13 Jan. 2014, www.theguardian.com/science/sifting-the-evidence/2014/jan/13/demystifying-detox-can-yoga-really-cleanse-the-liver.

"Spine Anatomy, Anatomy of the Human Spine." Edited by Tonya Hines, Mayfieldclinic.com, 10 Mar. 2017, mayfieldclinic.com/pe-anatspine.htm.

Tanenbaum, Sharon. "Increase Your Flexibility and Improve Your Life." Real Simple, www.realsimple.com/health/fitness-exercise/stretching-yoga/increase-flexibility-improve-life/.

"What Are We Really Saying With Namaste?" YogaDork, 27 July 2015, yogadork.com/2015/07/27/what-are-we-really-saying-with-namaste/.

"Yoga Meditation: Relaxation Before Meditation." Yoga Meditation, www.swamij.com/relaxation.htm.

"Yoga: What You Need To Know." Edited by Inna Belfer and David Shurtleff, National Center for Complementary and Integrative Health, U.S.

Department of Health and Human Services, 2018, www.nccih.nih.gov/
health/yoga-what-you-need-to-know.

CPSIA information can be obtained
at www.ICGtesting.com
Printed in the USA
LVHW031703080121
675851LV00002B/130